EXAMINATION OF THE SMALL INTESTINE
BY MEANS OF
DUODENAL INTUBATION

EXAMINATION
OF THE SMALL INTESTINE
BY MEANS OF
DUODENAL INTUBATION

J. L. SELLINK M. D.

H. E. STENFERT KROESE N.V. / LEIDEN 1971

Copyright 1971 by H. E. Stenfert Kroese N.V., Pieterskerkhof 38, P.O. Box 33,
Leiden, The Netherlands

Published simultaneously

in Japan by IGAKU SHOIN Ltd, 1-28-36 Hongo Bunkyo-Ku, Tokyo, Japan

Library of congress catalog card number 74-175454

ISBN 978-90-207-0297-2   ISBN 978-94-015-7185-2 (eBook)
DOI 10.1007/978-94-015-7185-2

CONTENTS

This study was performed in the Department of Radiology (Head: Prof. Dr. J. R. von Ronnen) of the Leiden University Hospital, The Netherlands.

Patients: Department of Gastroenterology (Head: Dr. A. J. Ch. Haex), and Department of Surgery (Head: Prof. Dr. M. Vink), Leiden University Hospital.

Drawings prepared by Mrs. J. J. M. de Vries-Jagersma and the author.

Photographs by M. G. Popkes and C. Th. Ruygrok, Department of Radiology, Leiden University Hospital.

Translation by Mrs. G. P. Bieger-Smith, Leiden.

I
INTRODUCTION

Our knowledge of the diseases of the small intestine has increased greatly since the second world war. The advances made in the auxiliary sciences, in particular biochemistry and histology, are mainly responsible and have led to their increased importance in this field.

It is unfortunate that although radiology also contributed new understanding, it has not been able to match the progress of the other sciences. In spite of the advancements made in, for instance, vascular examination, radiology has experienced a relative decrease in its importance to the differential diagnosis of the diseases of the small intestine. The main reason for this is that radiology can only offer an extremely modest contribution to the differentiation between the many diseases with the malabsorption syndrome. In a number of cases, radiological differential diagnosis is in principle not possible because there are only histological and biochemical abnormalities of the mucous membrane of the small intestine without macroscopic abnormalities. There remain however many diseases with malabsorption for which a morphological examination can be highly valuable. This applies for:

1. diseases with gross anatomical abnormalities:
    anastomoses, fistulae, blind loops;
    strictures, adhesions;
    diverticula.
2. diseases with local, usually rather gross mucosal abnormalities:
    leukemia, Hodgkin's disease, lymphosarcoma;
    intra-mural bleeding;
    local edema due to venous congestion (e.g. thrombosis) or lymphatic obstruction (irradiation treatment).
3. diseases with more general mucosal abnormalities:
    edema due to: lymphangiectasis,
                  allergic reactions,
                  protein-losing enteropathy;
    amyloidosis, Whipple's disease, scleroderma.

For some of these diseases, the radiologist is the only one who can provide the correct diagnosis. However, with the conventional methods of examination still in use, he often cannot even make a differential diagnosis and must suffice with the report that malabsorption probably exists. This opinion is based on the observation of flocculation (p. 20) as well as the eventual disintegration into segment clumps (p. 24) of the barium meal in the small intestine. This conclusion incidentally is seldom important since the referring specialist is usually already aware of the malabsorption syndrome on the basis of other evidence. As soon as flocculation occurs, every morphological evaluation of the small intestine becomes impossible, because there is no longer any relationship between the boundaries of the contrast spots and those of the intestinal mucous membrane (fig. 3). The flocculation is usually irreversible and the flocculi continue to grow in size until segments are formed. In addition, when the rate of transit of the contrast fluid through the small intestine is slow, this clump formation is further promoted in the distal ileum by the absorption of fluids from the intestine. In the colon, segmentation (p. 27) of the barium column is the natural end of every normal passage through the small intestine. When various methods of examination as well as the results obtained with diverse brands of contrast media are observed, it then becomes apparent that the development of flocculation is also highly dependent upon both of these factors. As a result, one radiologist will observe flocculation frequently and the other only when there is a serious malabsorption. The highly illogical situation then arises that a radiologist can only interpret the small bowel examination of a colleague to a limited degree. Even if there are signs of a pronounced and relatively early flocculation on the x-ray film of a patient with a known malabsorption, he will not be able to express his opinion about the severity of this malabsorption. It is therefore obvious that in the roentgenologic findings an observed flocculation and segmentation must be reported such that faulty conclusions will not be drawn. In fact, this means that each radiologist builds up experience exclusively for himself based on the use of one specific contrast medium for one specific method of examination; this experience cannot be transferred to someone else. Should he change one or both of these aspects, then he has lost his experience in this respect and he must start again.

The radiological diagnosis of tumors in the small intestine is almost as difficult as the differentiation between diseases with the malabsorption syndrome. In 1938 this caused insurmountable difficulties (33) in cases without any obstruction and even today the radiologist seldom finds a tumor in the small intestine of a patient with limited clinical symptoms.

According to various articles, 1.5 to 6.5 per cent of the total number of tumors in the digestive tract are localized in the small intestine (146, 33). Although there are more malignant tumors in the stomach and more benign tumors in the colon, in the small intestine both types appear with approximately the same frequency (77). It is fortunate that most of the tumors are located in the duodenum and in the distal part of the ileum because in fact these two areas are the most accessible for unimpeded radiological examination. The fact that many tumors in the remaining parts of the small intestine are never diagnosed is however usually due to the technical execution of the examination and not the flocculation of the contrast medium. An additional drawback is that many radiologists do not take enough exposures of the small intestine and during the examination, the films are studied insufficiently or not at all. Although it is normal to take many spot films during fluoroscopy of the stomach and colon, this is usually not done for the much longer small intestine.

The difficulties encountered in locating smaller abnormalities in the mid-portion of the small intestine are demonstrated by the fact that the radiologist seldom finds a Meckel's diverticulum while a study of autopsy material has shown that this occurs in 2 per cent of the deceased.

For as long as the radiological examination of the small intestine has existed, now almost 70 years, the transit time has been included in the roentgenological report. The transit time however appears to be highly dependent upon many factors, including not only the pyloric function but also the quantity, the caloric value, the temperature and the method of administration of the contrast medium.

When RIEDER (180) introduced his standard 'meal' at the beginning of the century, this meal was in general use and recording the transit time was probably useful. This harmony however did not last very long because the method of examination and the use of contrast media later became highly diversified. It is therefore not surprising that the average transit time reported between 1930 and 1950 by prominent radiologists varied between 2 and 5 hours with extreme values of 1 and 8 hours (124). From the above, it is obvious that including these values on x-ray films and in reports is exceedingly unimportant today. It would probably be better to omit them since they can lead to incorrect conclusions.

In principle, the radiologist can also carry out a functional examination of the small intestine; until now however only a few attempts have been made in this direction. The difficulties in this field are still enormous so that realization of this type of examination will require more advanced experimentation. A condition for a functional examination is in any event a contrast meal with caloric value, obtained by adding nutrients. Unfortunately the stability (p. 27) of the contrast media now available is inadequate since all additives with caloric value cause flocculation.

Even in 1958 PYGOTT wrote that a follow-through examination of the small bowel has no value and as a routine study cannot be justified (172). Since then there has been little change; for many radiologists the examination of the small intestine is a stepchild, for others a problem child.

There has long been agreement about the best way to carry out examinations of the upper gastro-intestinal tract and the colon, but a good examination technique without disadvantages does not yet seem to exist for the small intestine. A contrast medium which meets all requirements and which is without any doubt the best also does not exist. It is therefore not surprising that the examination of the small intestine has fallen into disrepute and is often not carried out in the best possible manner. In The Netherlands even the cost reimbursement tariff of the health service reflects this situation, because it is by far not enough to cover the actual costs of an adequate roentgenological examination.

AIMS

The aim of this study is to attempt to bring about an improvement in the unsatisfactory results of the radiological examination of the small intestine. These poor results can be blamed on the method of examination or the contrast medium used, or may be even both. In the chapters to follow, an attempt will be made to investigate this problem further by considering all factors involved in the radiological examination of the small intestine.

II
HISTORY*

Within six months after the discovery of x-rays by WILHELM CONRAD RÖNTGEN in December 1895, WEGELE had localized the human stomach by inserting a tube containing a metal wire. HEMMETER used a tube to introduce lead acetate into the stomach after first testing this procedure on mice. Also in 1896, WALTER CANNON of Boston introduced a mixture of bread and bismuth** into the beak of a goose and using the fluoroscope, studied the mechanism of deglutition. In 1897, he used the same contrast medium to observe the peristaltic movements of the stomach of a cat. In the same year, BOAS and LEVY-DORN published their method for the examination of the human stomach. As contrast medium, they used bismuth nitrate packaged in capsules of gelatin and cellulose. In France, ROUX and BALTHAZARD also studied the human stomach; they used the same contrast medium but made a pap of water and syrup. In Germany fluoroscopic studies of the human esophagus were made using a 5 per cent suspension of bismuth in water. The bismuth nitrate is highly poisonous in large quantities and was quickly replaced by bismuth carbonate. In 1898, RIEDER administered the bismuth in the form of tablets or cookies; HOLZKNECHT made a paste with lactose in 1900 and several years later, a solution of 10 g bismuth with a teaspoon of lactose in 50 ml water.

The quality of the x-ray films left a great deal to be desired; tube current and tube voltage were very low so that exposure times occasionally lasted minutes.

Since they also wished to document the results of fluoroscopy, the images were quickly drawn by hand during the examination.

The examination of the digestive tract was only carried out incidentally and was predominantly functional in character. Measured by our modern standards, the requirements set were not high; interest was centered mainly on the stomach and the rate at which it emptied. Only very gross morphological abnormalities could be shown indirectly, such as a cardiospasm, an almost complete stenosis due to tumor growth or a hourglass stomach. For example, HOLZKNECHT (90) based a diagnosis of pylorus carcinoma on the following symptoms:

bismuth residual after 6 hours,
normal stomach shadow,
capsule intact after 5 hours.

and a diagnosis of gastric ulcer on:

small bismuth residual after 6 hours,
normal stomach shadow,
localized tenderness during palpation.

---

* From: GIANTURCO C. (68); HOLZKNECHT G. (90); RIGLER and WEINER in: *Alimentary tract roentgenology* (131); KNOX R. (101); LEDOUX-LEBARD G. (116).
** In earlier publications it is not always possible to discover which bismuthsalt was used.

However not until 1904 did the examination of the digestive tract find greater acceptance due to the pioneering publication by RIEDER (180). He described in great detail the examination of the stomach in fixed standard positions and listed the times when the subsequent transit pictures of the intestine should be made. He also introduced a standard meal for the examination, called Rieder gruel, which consisted of a mixture of 200 g semolina pap and 30 g bismuth. In this publication, RIEDER also demonstrated that the use of larger quantities of bismuth as contrast medium was not detrimental. In addition he listed several diagnostic criteria which, for the small intestine, were restricted to the rate of transit and signs of obstruction. Study of the mucous membrane was not possible; the duodenum could only be recognized by its shape. Around the jejunum and ileum, loops could not even be distinguished, so that these parts of the small intestine received no further attention.

Later RIEDER replaced his thick gruel with a suspension of 30 g bismuth in buttermilk, a mixture which was used until the twenties. This resulted in an improvement in the image quality, but satisfactory images of the ileum could still not be obtained. RIEDER therefore believed that it was better to carry out a retrograde examination of the ileum using a colon enema. In the meantime, differential diagnosis had been extended to include the diagnosis of tuberculosis which could be suspected if there were obstructions in the small intestine. Whether or not the appendix filled during a small intestinal passage also became a consideration of some significance.

In general there seems to have been a tendency to increase the bismuth content of the contrast meal and to replace food by water. One example is JOLLASSE's recipe of 1907: (98) he mixed 30 g bismuth with 15 g sugar and some water as needed. JOLLASSE had observed that the administration of a physiological contrast meal served no purpose since the bismuth settles and remains behind after the food has left the stomach. He was certainly one of the first to realize that the uppermost fluid level seen fluoroscopically during a stomach examination usually represents the food mixture. Before his publication this fluid level was always attributed to secretion due to PAWLOW's response. Apparently there was an exaggerated idea of the flavor of and the appetite aroused by the contrast meal. JOLLASSE saw that during the examination of the stomach, the level of the bismuth decreased but the contrast intensity increased. The samples which he obtained from the fluid levels with a tube confirmed his opinions.

In 1907 KAESTLE also considered the problem of sedimentation; his extensive publication is the oldest on this subject (100). He thought that this problem would not exist for a gastrointestinal examination because a good flour pap causes practically no sedimentation (p. 18). For the colon examination, on the other hand, bismuth was mixed with water only and sedimentation was very troublesome. He combatted this phenomenon by adding 5 parts bolus alba for each part bismuth to the contrast fluid. The composition of the resulting mixture, which was suited for eventual oral use, was as follows:

30 g bismuth carbonate,
150 g bolus alba,
300 ml water.

KAESTLE also tried to overcome sedimentation by adding tragacanth or arabic gum to the contrast fluid but the results were not satisfactory.

It is interesting to note the ideas prevalent at that time about the origin of the segmentation of the contrast column in the small intestine. It was believed that the stiffness of the 'bismuth sausage' was so great that it broke into fragments of necessity since otherwise the curves in the small intestinal loops could not be passed.

It is not known exactly how bismuth came to be chosen as the contrast medium; even in 1902 CANNON had mentioned that in addition to bismuth, barium could also be used. CANNON however chose bismuth powder on purpose because he knew that it could be obtained in a purer form than barium powder. The preparation of pure barium powder was not found at that time in the American pharmacopeia; bismuth powder on the other hand was listed.

KAESTLE, who was not happy with the pronounced tendency of bismuth toward sedimentation, also searched for other contrast media. He considered however only those elements with an atomic number greater than that of bismuth, such as thorium and uranium. These two elements of course could not be considered because of their rareness and high prices. At that time their radioactive properties were still unknown. Collargol, a soluble silver compound could not be satisfactorily used in the amounts considered safe because of the lack in contrast. He probably did not test barium, which is slightly lighter than bismuth, for the following reasons:

The contrast intensity of the films and fluoroscopic images obtained with bismuth was so low that a decrease could not be tolerated. In fact since only 30 g bismuth was used for approximately 300 ml contrast medium, the specific gravity of the mixture could not have been much higher than 1.1. Presumably because he had so little experience with barium, he did not dare use 30 g, thus a higher volume dosage. However at a radiological congress in 1910, KRAUSE of Bonn propagated the use of barium as a contrast medium. In spite of the fact that barium has the advantage of costing much less than bismuth, he did not succeed in introducing barium. Less than a year later however, his compatriots BACHEM and GÜNTHER were successful; they also suggested that chemically barium sulfate can be made purer than bismuth salts. Nevertheless bismuth was still preferred as contrast medium, certainly after publications appeared about the detrimental side-effects of barium, probably resulting from impurities. Not until the first world war did barium completely replace bismuth. Bismuth was necessary for the war industry and was therefore very scarce and expensive. After this war, bismuth was essentially no longer in use; positive experience in the use of barium had been gained in the meantime.

It was still common practice to administer a physiological food mixture, now however mixed with barium instead of bismuth. For example, we can find many recipes of this type in HOLZKNECHT's handbook dating from 1931. Several are listed below; together they also demonstrate that at that time a standard contrast meal no longer existed.

1. universal contrast medium:
   40–80 g $BaSO_4$ in 500 ml water.
   Stir until just before use to prevent sedimentation.
2. barium pap:
   100–150 g $BaSO_4$,
   3–4 tablespoons semolina,
   250 ml water.
3. paste suitable for prolonged storage:
   mixture of equal parts of $BaSO_4$ and paraffin oil.
4. barium pap of Schlesinger:
   180 g $BaSO_4$,
   20 g chocolate powder,
   3 g mondamine,
   250 ml water.
5. barium pap of Günther:
   150 g $BaSO_4$,
   150 g mondamine,
   20 g cocoa,
   15 g sugar,
   500 ml water.
6. paste of Schwarz:
   mixture of barium and apricot jam.
7. paste of Schlesinger:
   mixture of 80 g barium and 6 teaspoons applesauce.
8. for infants:
   mixture of barium and mother's milk.
9. for examination of the colon:
   100 g bismuth in 1000 ml water.

To obtain films of the digestive tract, HOLZKNECHT recommended a voltage of 55–60 kV, although the maximum obtainable tube voltage was 80–90 kV. The tube current was 30–40 mA; the exposure times were on the order of several seconds. Several clinics, including the Leiden University Hospital, preferred pictures which are interpreted more easily over the use of a physiological contrast medium, but they remained a minority until the second world war.

Only after CROHN's article in 1932 (37) on stenosing ileitis not caused by tuberculosis and the article by SNELL and CAMP (198) about chronic idiopathic steatorrhea was the interest in small bowel examination awakened. There were still some however who failed to see any point in the radiological examination of the small intestine. Even in 1937, WELTZ (214) wrote that for the small intestine morphological diagnosis is in principle impossible in contrast to functional diagnosis. It is in any event likely that his films were difficult to read because he used a calory-rich contrast meal. In 1932, COLE's co-workers (36) wrote that the ileum could only be identified by segmentation, and the jejunum by flocculation.

PRÉVÔT (171) did not agree; since more is known about the anatomy of the small intestine than the physiology, he considered a morphological evaluation more feasible than a physiological evaluation. He believed that the differences between the mucosal pattern on an x-ray film and on the autopsy table must be ascribed to the influence of tone and peristalsis. The fact that his patients underwent laxation before the passage examination in order to prevent mixture of the contrast medium with the bowel contents proves that he was far ahead of his times.

Because it was necessary to reject bismuth as a contrast medium, the beginning of the first world war actually concluded a phase in the development of the examination of the small intestine.

About 1940, again at the beginning of a world war, another period in this development was closed. The differential diagnoses at that time included the following diseases: polyposis, diverticula, tuberculosis, regional ileitis, leukemia infiltrations and M. Hodgkin (169).

Up until 1940 development of the radiological examination of the small intestine proceeded slowly; this can certainly be attributed to the limited detail reproduced by the contrast fluids used up to that time. The common practice of mixing barium with food was another important factor contributing to this lack of detail. During the second world war, most radiologists could not obtain the barium preparations they were used to. It then became necessary to use another brand or to prepare a suspension themselves. For many radiologists this resulted in the discovery that the characteristics of the diverse barium preparations vary greatly. They were therefore encouraged to try to improve the composition of the contrast medium. This resulted in a considerable improvement in the detail reproduced which in turn led to an expansion of the differential diagnosis.

A second important factor in the further development of the examination of the small bowel since 1940 was the appearance of numerous publications by ROSS GOLDEN. As no other, this radiologist studied the diseases of the small intestine and their radiological recognition. Only the conventional method of examination and the equally conventional contrast medium used at the height of his career limited the enormous significance of this man for the development of the radiological examination of the small intestine. ROSS GOLDEN can certainly be called the founder of modern differential diagnosis of the small bowel. His work has stimulated others to greater activity and intensive study of all aspects which might be important for a better understanding of the roentgenological pictures of the small intestine. These studies encompass anatomy, physiology, composition of the contrast medium and the method of examination. In the following chapters, these subjects will each be discussed separately.

III
ANATOMY

More important for a correct interpretation of the pictures obtained than for the technical execution of the examination is a thorough knowledge of the anatomical structure of the wall of the small intestine. It is however difficult to differentiate between examination and interpretation, at least when the radiologist is actively involved in both as is the case for gastric and colon examinations.

For 90 per cent of the patients, the jejunum is located in the left upper quadrant and the ileum in the right lower quadrant of the abdomen; according to ZIMMER, a small convolution usually lies in the middle and forms the transition between these two intestinal sections (223). The lack of this 'intermediate convolution' may be the most frequent anomaly. Now and then we are confronted with an inversion of the small intestine; the jejunum then lies in the right upper quadrant of the abdomen and the ileum in the middle or in the left lower quadrant. Quite rare are the cases of a total stomach-intestine inversion or an anomaly whereby the jejunum lies in the middle of the upper abdomen, the ileum in the middle of the lower abdomen and the stomach and cecum completely to the left.

The wall of the small intestine consists of the following layers, starting from the outside:

1. the serosa,
2. the tunica muscularis, which consists of an outer longitudinal layer and an inner circular layer,
3. the submucosa, which contains many blood and lymphatic vessels in a loose connective tissue so that the tunica muscularis can move freely with respect to:
4. the mucosa; this layer is made up of three parts:
   a. the muscularis mucosa which, like the tunica muscularis, consists of an outer longitudinal layer and an inner circular layer. The muscular strands of this inner circular layer extend into the folds of Kerkring and some even extend through the tunica propria into the villi which cover the surface of the mucosa. The villi vary in number from 10 to 40 per mm^2; they are 0.2–1 mm high and have a centrally located, blind ended lymphatic vessel. Between the villi are the crypts of Lieberkühn.
   b. the tunica propria, like the submucosa, consists of a loose connective tissue containing blood and lymphatic vessels as well as nerve fibers. Occasionally conglomerates of lymphocytes are found in this layer.
   c. a layer of simple columnar epithelial cells which can move freely with respect to the tunica propria. The surface of each epithelial cell is covered with hundreds of microvilli (200).

The folds of Kerkring begin 3–5 cm beyond the pylorus; in the proximal part of the jejunum, they are 3–6 mm high and 1–3 mm apart. Distally the folds are less high and they become more widely separated. The thickness of the folds is 1–2 mm in both the jejunum and the ileum; in the ileum however they tend to lie in a more longitudinal direction. During a contraction, the folds in the jejunum also extend in a more longitudinal direction (118).

In addition, the number and height of the villi decreases in the distal direction. WILSON computed mathematically that for a length of small intestine of 5.5 m, the surface of the mucosa is about 2.2 m² (215). If we assume an average diameter of 2 cm for the lumen, then the folds of Kerkring and the villi increase the surface of the mucosa more than 6 times, more in the jejunum and less in the ileum. The microvilli also increase the surface of the epithelial cells at least 15 times (200). The total increase in the surface due to the folds, villi and microvilli can therefore be estimated as 100 times.

The intramural nervous system of the intestinal wall is very complicated; the histological handbooks (BLOOM and FAWCETT, HAM, BUCHER and STÖHR) describe 4 systems:

1. the subserosal plexus,
2. the myenteric plexus of Auerbach, which lies between the circular and longitudinal layers of the muscle coat,
3. the plexus muscularis profundus in the circular muscular layer,
4. the submucosal plexus of Meissner which consists of several layers of interconnected fiber networks. The most important layer lies close to the muscularis mucosa. Some fibers from this layer extend to the muscularis mucosa and others continue through the tunica propria to the villi, glands and epithelial cells. There is also a layer close to the inner circular muscular layer of the tunica muscularis.

The anatomy of the wall of the small intestine is shown schematically in fig. 1.

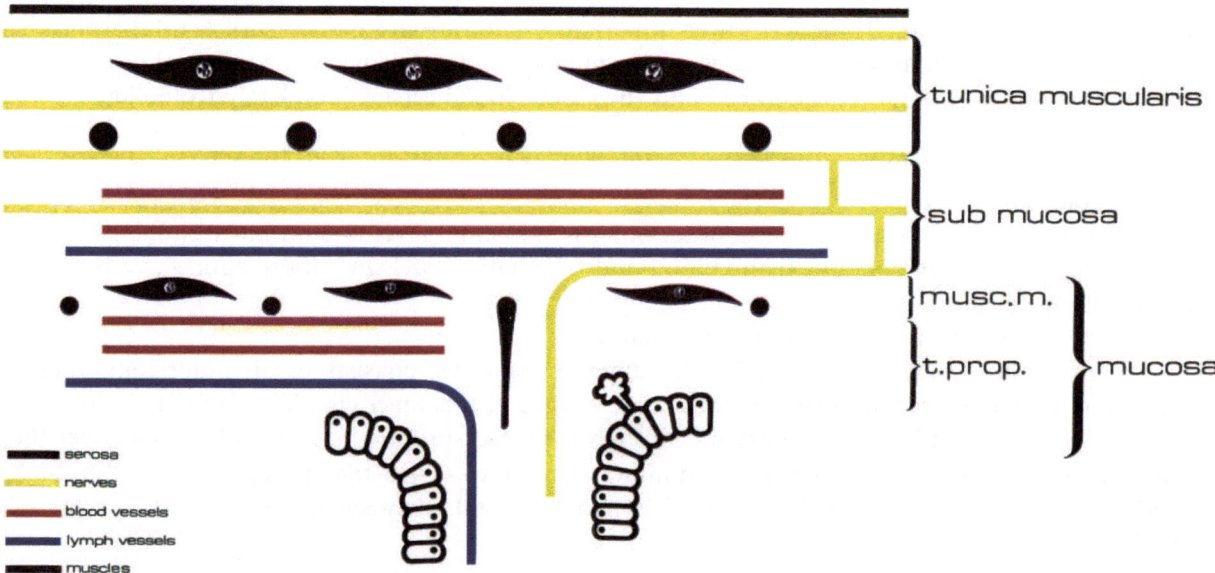

Fig. 1
Schematical cross-section of intestinal wall

Although several studies have been published concerning the length of the small intestine, the definitive answer has yet to be found. Most handbooks list values varying between 5 and 7 meters and the small intestine is assumed to be $\frac{3}{5}$ of the total length of the digestive tract. It is known that the length of the small intestine is highly dependent upon the tone, so that the results of measurements taken post-mortem or under anaesthesia will be too high.

Some authors state that an asthenic will have a slightly longer small intestine than a pycnic. In fact for pycnic patients we have almost never had problems of superposition of a convolution of ileum loops in the small pelvis. A length of 12 m may not be unusual for American negroes and in India.

X-ray films of the small intestine show that occasionally an individual variation can be enormous. However when several measurements of the same patient are taken, the results appear to differ by only 10 per cent at the most (87). UNDERHILL (209) obtained post-mortem values of 4.7–9.7 m for an average length of 6.9 m. Unfortunately she took some measurements several hours after death and others after the body had been stored for several days.

HIRSCH et al. (87) report that shortly after death contraction of the smooth musculature causes the intestine to shorten; autolysis later causes a renewed increase in length. They took measurements in vivo by having patients swallow a rubber tube 3.5 mm in diameter; their values then varied between 220 and 270 cm from mouth to anus. When they used a tube 2 mm in diameter, the results were 400–540 cm, thus considerably longer. Post-mortem however these values turned out to be 800–900 cm! The shortening of the intestine around an ingested tube is called the 'telescope effect'.

The distance from nose or mouth to the duodeno-jejunal flexure varies only slightly; a length of 90 cm! is assumed here. The colon length varies between 100 and 150 cm. These studies have clearly shown that the tone of the musculature of the intestinal wall influences not only the diameter but also the length of the small intestine; because of these two factors, the tone therefore determines to an important degree the extent of superposition.

For the jejunum, the diameter is normally assumed to be 2.5–3 cm and for the ileum, 2–2.5 cm. Values have also been reported of 1 and 0.5 inch respectively, which are probably a closer approximation of the diameter in vivo.

The mucosal pattern can, depending upon the state of contraction or dilatation, also show very pronounced changes. SLOAN (197) demonstrated this very clearly.

Until the second world war, it was assumed that the mucosa and the nervous system of the intestinal wall of infants were still markedly underdeveloped, because for the first 3–6 months mucosal patterns were never seen on the x-ray films, not even in the duodenum. The appearance of a baby's small intestine on the x-ray films at that time was strikingly similar to that of an adult with a severe malabsorption or 'deficiency state' (less stable contrast medium and therefore flocculation caused by mucin and lactic acid). It was assumed that this deficiency state must be ascribed to damaged nerve cells since the pathologist found vacuolar degeneration in these cells. The x-ray films often showed flattening or even disappearance of the relief of the mucosal folds (GOLDEN 74).

BOUSLOG (20, 21) and WELTZ (214) were also not able to observe mucosal patterns on the x-ray films of infants but their studies had shown that the mucosal folds are more highly developed both absolutely and relatively than those of an adult and are even present in the third fetal month. The folds are however thinner and not as high. Vascularization and cell-richness are pronounced in the mucosa. The submucosa is smaller than that of an adult so that the muscularis, the mucosa and the submucosa of an infant are all of approximately equal thickness. The relative underdevelopment of the muscularis, also in the mucosa, could cause the mucosal folds to be flattened completely by the barium column.

All x-ray films published before the second world war show only a pronounced segmentation of the barium column, even in the duodenum. In general therefore one suspects that these examinations were in vain and that the conclusions were probably incorrect more often than correct.

Although the composition of many contrast media has been greatly improved, articles still appear today reporting that mucosal patterns cannot be observed until the infant is several months old. It is also stated however that no conclusions may be drawn from this fact.

IV
PHYSIOLOGY

Introduction

It is common to feel that one is less able to influence the course of a transit examination than that of a colon or gastro-duodenal examination.

If an improvement in the results is desired, it is necessary to ascertain where, when and how to intervene. It is obvious that for this purpose, some fundamental knowledge of several important physiological aspects is required. Therefore the following factors shall be discussed separately:

1. innervation of the small intestine,
2. tone and peristalsis,
3. function of the pyloric muscle,
4. influence of nutrients on gastric emptying time and rate of transit through the small intestine,
5. influence of the volume of the contrast meal on the gastric emptying time,
6. effect of the absorption of fluids from the contrast column in the distal ileum,
7. obstructions in the small intestine.

1. Innervation of the small intestine

The parasympathetic innervation of the small intestine occurs via the celiac ganglion by fibers of the right vagus nerve. Cutting the vagus causes a decrease in the motility of the small intestine and therefore a reduced rate of transit. The sympathetic innervation occurs via the splanchnic nerves. The fibers of both systems lie in the mesentery and belong to the central nervous system.

The intramural autonomic nervous system is exceedingly important for the small intestine. It consists of the plexus of Auerbach in the tunica muscularis and the plexus of Meissner in the submucosa (see fig. 1).

LOEWI (1921) and DALE (1929) showed that when the parasympathetic nerves are stimulated, acetylcholine is produced; in 1933 CANNON demonstrated that stimulation of the sympathetic nerves produces adrenin which has the same effect as adrenalin. Acetylcholine plays an important role in the transmission of nervous impulses; it is not soluble in fat and cannot pass through the lipoidal membranes of the nerve fibers. Acetylcholine causes contraction of the muscle fibers. Termination of this contraction is caused by the repeated inactivation of acetylcholine by the enzyme acetylcholinesterase. This enzyme can be inactivated by neostigmine; when this occurs, the breakdown of acetylcholine is retarded and the state of contraction or the tone lasts longer. This heightened tone causes an enhancement of the peristalsis, especially in the jejunum. As a result, the jejunum resembles the ileum more closely: the diameter decreases and the folds extend in a more longitudinal direction.

The intensification of peristalsis produced by neostigmine or prostigmin is used in intravenous pyelography to remove troublesome small gas bubbles from the small intestine. It is well-known that air in the small intestine moves so fast in the distal direction that it takes only several minutes to travel from the stomach to the cecum. Large gas bubbles generally remove themselves from the digestive tract since they cause sufficient stretching of the intestinal wall to induce peristaltic contractions (126).

The effect of prostigmin is cancelled by atropine. Neostigmine has no effect on patients with sprue; it is tentatively assumed that this is due to a disturbed functioning of the nerve cells. In this respect the role of vitamin B deficiencies is still unknown.

2. Tone and peristalsis

In 1923, FORSSELL (53) showed that the movements of the muscularis mucosae are independent and not, as was generally assumed, dependent upon contractions of the tunica muscularis. Using x-ray films and autopsy material, he observed that a given intestinal segment with a lumen of a specific diameter displays highly divergent mucosal patterns. He assumed that the movements of the muscularis mucosae might fulfill an important role in the digestion of food.

In 1922, the physiologists KING and ARNOLD (103) made similar observations but it is not clear whether FORSSELL was aware of this. They noted that mechanical stimulation of the ends of the villi only caused contractions of the stimulated villi, usually once but occasionally several times in succession. Stimulation at the base of the villi caused contractions of the villi as a group. The mucosa appeared to be stimulated not only locally but also via the splanchnic nerves. The plexus of Meissner probably regulates only the tone. Stimulation of the muscularis mucosae is not possible via the plexus of Auerbach; however stimulation of the mucosa does cause a relaxation of the tone of the tunica muscularis, followed by a recovery. The rate of this recovery increases as the stimulation is intensified. Physiologically, mechanical stimulation by the food mass is the most important factor causing contractions of the tunica muscularis. The reflex mechanism for these peristaltic waves is via the plexus of Auerbach and it will only respond to stimulation of this plexus (103). Peristaltic waves of the tunica muscularis are characterized by relaxation before and contraction behind the area stimulated. Although similar in motion to milking, the mechanism involved is not known precisely since it is highly complicated (118). The longitudinal fibers shorten behind the advancing circular contractions. The frequency of the peristaltic waves is approximately 1 per sec. In the case of hypermotility, this frequency increases only slightly, but the contractions clearly become more pronounced. There are fewer peristaltic contractions in the ileum than in the jejunum and the latent period between stimulation and contraction is the longest in the distal part of the small intestine. In addition, the movements of the villi decrease in the distal direction. This gradual decrease in diverse vital functions from proximal to distal is called the 'metabolic gradient' (p. 58).

Normally peristaltic contractions should not occur in the ileum; they are seen however when there is an increased excitability of the intestine or a lowered stimulus threshold. The ileum is characterized by segmentation moving in the aboral direction; the intestinal contents are constricted at regular intervals and divided up into the so-called 'segments of Cannon' (119).

Nicotine and stimulation of the vagus influence the tunica muscularis but not the muscularis mucosae (103). The development of the movements of the mucosa appears to be highly dependent upon a good blood supply (103, 75). ABBOTT and PENDERGRASS (1) found that when morphine is administered directly into the duodenum, there is a pronounced increase in the tone which decreases in the distal direction. 15 to 20 minutes later, the tone decreases; it is once again the greatest in the duodenum and decreases in the distal direction. Using a double balloon to register the change in the pressure in the small intestine, they observed that the motility is highly dependent upon the differences in tone and that the intensity of the peristaltic waves increases with an increase in the tone of the intestinal wall. LENZ and KREPPEL (120) studied the influence of prostigmin, pilocarpine and arecoline on the motility of the small intestine of a cat, which is structured similar to that of man. The movements of the contrast column were filmed. After prostigmin was injected, the tone increased and the Cannon constrictions became more pronounced and more frequent; the number of peristaltic contractions also increased. The prostigmin was ineffective 9 minutes later and hypotonia occurred.

The results with pilocarpine and arecoline were similar but more pronounced. In particular pilocarpine induced a greater secretion production so that dilution of the contrast medium was greater than with prostigmin. The mucosal folds were clearly broadened; autopsy showed that this was due to edema. Overdosage of prostigmin and arecoline caused spasms and dyskinesia; peristaltic waves no longer occurred. An overdosage of pilocarpine did not cause dyskinesia, but there was such heavy secretion and edematous swelling of the mucous membrane that peristaltic waves were no longer possible mechanically.

In 1931, PANSDORF had already observed swelling of the folds of Kerkring caused by pilocarpine in 18 healthy persons. The effect of these 3 substances, called the muscarine effect, is similar to that of postganglionic sympathetic stimulation and can be neutralized by atropine. Pilocarpine and arecoline act directly on the smooth musculature; prostigmin acts on cholinesterase.

GERSHON-COHEN, SHAY and FELS (65) found that barium test meals cooled to 35–40° F left the stomach sooner and (therefore) passed through the small intestine more quickly than contrast meals heated up to 140–145° F. The mechanism of this accelerated gastric emptying and rapid transit due to temperature decrease is not known. The supposition that it is due to insufficient digestion and absorption resulting from decreased secretion is speculative. Gastric secretion decreases markedly when the gastric contents are cold; however when the gastric contents are warm, secretion increases to only slightly above the norm. For cold gastric contents, secretion returns to normal more rapidly than the increase in the temperature of the gastric contents suggests.

3. Function of the pyloric muscle

Ever since 1907, it has been known that isotonic solutions leave the stomach faster than hypotonic or hypertonic solutions (123). Only small amounts of hypertonic solutions pass through the pylorus to the duodenum where as a result they quickly become isotonic. At the same time, the stomach also attempts to make the hypertonic solution isotonic by fluid secretion. Using HCl and Na_2CO_3, SHAY and GERSHON-COHEN demonstrated that the responses of the stomach and the pylorus are the same, whether the hypertonic solution is administered into the stomach or directly into the duodenum by intubation (190). JOHNSTON and RAVDIN (97) used glucose-barium on dogs with gastric resections to demonstrate that severe contractions of the small intestine compensate to some extent for the absence of the pylorus. They also observed this for patients.

In spite of the regulatory effect of stomach and pylorus, it is possible to introduce a hypertonic solution orally into the duodenum, where it becomes isotonic due to the attraction of fluids (97). The resulting increase in volume causes the intestinal wall to stretch which in turn causes a more active peristalsis. This peristalsis can vary greatly for the same tone. For a rapid increase in pressure in the testinal lumen, the stimulus threshold for the development of peristaltic waves is lower than for a slow increase in pressure. The stimulus threshold is also lower for an increased tone than for a decreased tone (38). For an exceptionally large increase in pressure or pronounced stretching of the intestinal wall, which physiologically probably do not occur, an inhibition of the motility develops after a latent period of 2–3 seconds. This entero-intestinal 'inhibitory reflex' (219) develops more rapidly as the stretching or pressure as well as the length of the intestinal segment involved increases.

Another well-known fact is that fear and emotions influence the small intestine by causing an increase in tone and an enhancement of the peristalsis. Because there is not enough time for the absorption of fluids, diarrhea develops. The opening and closing of the pylorus is a very complicated mechanism which is only partially understood. Almost everyone who has studied this mechanism has found that a peristaltic wave in the stomach is not necessarily followed by relaxation of the pylorus.

In addition to the caloric value of the gastric and duodenal contents, osmosis and pH also play an important role (66, 178, 190). GERSHON-COHEN et al. (66) showed that a hypotonic solution leaves the stomach almost as fast as an isotonic solution. However when these solutions are introduced directly into the duodenum, then the hypotonic solution causes the pylorus to remain closed until isotonicity is achieved. A solution becomes isotonic much faster in the duodenum than in the stomach where it results from an increase in the salt content of the secreted gastric juice. The contents of the duodenum are usually slightly acidic, depending upon the composition of the ingested food. It appears that prolonged closing of the pylorus is not caused by highly acidic contents alone; this also occurs when sodium bicarbonate is introduced via a tube causing the duodenal contents to become alkaline (35). This mechanism of duodenal neutralization is the most highly developed in hyperchlorhydria and the least in achlorhydria. The most sensitive reactions to tone and acidity occur in the proximal part of the duodenum and decrease in the distal direction (190).

For an empty stomach, the pylorus is relaxed which explains why the bulb is so often well filled immediately after administration of the first few mouthfuls of barium in a gastric examination. Shortly afterwards the pylorus closes; the latent period for this reaction is several seconds. The tone of the gastric musculature depends upon the conditions in the duodenum and is the stimulus for the development of peristaltic waves. These peristaltic waves are however not necessary for gastric emptying; the stomach can also empty if there is sufficient tone and an open pyloric canal. The pylorus is more relaxed in achlorhydria than when there is free acid in the stomach. If the other conditions remain the same, then the stomach empties faster in achlorhydria.

4. Influence of nutrients on gastric emptying time and rate of transit through the small intestine

The influence of nutrients on gastric emptying and transit through the small intestine can best be studied using carbohydrates. Glucose was chosen because it mixes easily with the contrast fluid and with it, the contrast fluid can easily be made hypertonic. Hypertonic gastric contents first become isotonic; during this process, the volume can increase considerably. For example, 215 ml of a 50 per cent glucose solution increases to more than 500 ml after 1 hour in the stomach (123); 100 ml of a 10 per cent glucose solution increases to 128 ml after 12 min. and 40 min. later, it is still 122 ml. When a 3.5 per cent glucose solution is administered orally, then 1 hour later the glucose concentration in the small intestine is 2.6 mg per 100 ml. If a 50 per cent glucose solution is used, this concentration is only 5.3 mg per 100 ml, a relatively small difference.

REYNOLDS et al. (178) compared the gastric emptying time for 33 children using 5 different mixtures of the contrast medium. They examined each child five times and found the values as shown in the table on page 16.

If we consider the fact that the high value of the 5th test is due to the greater amount administered, then we can conclude from the above that fat is the slowest to leave the stomach. This conclusion is in

Contrast medium:	Gastric emptying time:
1. 60 g Ba + 120 g water	1.9 hours
2. 60 g Ba + 120 g milk (2.33 per cent fat)	3.1 hours
3. 60 g Ba + 120 g cream (13.33 per cent fat)	4.8 hours
4. 60 g Ba + 90 g water + 30 g syrup	3.3 hours
5. 40 g Ba + 200 g water + 100 g protein	5.0 hours
(3.5 per cent fat, 7 per cent protein)	

agreement with that of MENVILLE and ANÉ (142) who carried out similar tests on adults and found that proteins and carbohydrates retard gastric emptying to the same extent, but fats considerably more. Fat was also the most important factor causing retarded transit through the small bowel.

Although a resection stomach empties faster than a normal stomach, here too the addition of nutrients to the contrast medium has a delaying effect. Because of the presence of glucose in the proximal part of the small intestine, enterogastrone is produced, a hormone which inhibits the peristalsis of the stomach. Similar mechanisms also exist for fat and possibly protein.

VAN LIERE et al. (123) introduced 50 ml of an indifferent mixture into the stomach of dogs who had first received an intravenous glucose injection. Autopsy showed that a half hour later this mixture had moved an average of 141 cm in the small intestine in contrast to 183 cm for the control group. The blood sugar was then 183 mg per cent versus 99 mg per cent for the control group. According to their report, the inhibitory influence of a high blood sugar concentration on the peristalsis of stomach and intestine has been known since 1924. A low blood sugar concentration on the other hand causes contractions of the stomach and a feeling of hunger.

5. Influence of the volume of the contrast meal on the gastric emptying time

HENDERSON (84) studied the gastric emptying time for 110 infants using specific amounts of contrast medium; he found values of 8–24 hours for a new-born child, 4–5 hours for a baby 2 weeks old and 2–3 hours for babies 3–4 months old. He therefore advised that the fasting period before examination of the baby should be longer than the usual 4 hours. He observed that 2/3 of the contrast medium leaves the stomach rather quickly but the remaining 1/3 takes considerably longer. He also saw that the stomach empties faster in a hanging position or a right lateral position and that good mucosal patterns can be obtained only under these conditions, sometimes even into the proximal ileum. He was not able to find an explanation for this observation.

Even the size of the meal influences the gastric emptying time. VAN LIERE et al. reported emptying times for 200 ml, 400 ml, and 600 ml in normal individuals. They found that 400 ml of a watery barium suspension took only 16.83 per cent instead of 100 per cent longer to leave the stomach than 200 ml; 600 ml took 38.33 per cent longer. The use of two decimal places suggests an accuracy in conflict with the small number of persons tested. It is also improbable that the second supplementary dosage of 200 ml took 38.33 — 2 × 16.83 = 4.67 per cent longer to leave the stomach than the first supplementary dosage of 200 ml. However the inaccuracies caused by these small numbers does not change the importance of their statistically significant observations (123). This phenomenon can only be explained by the greater supply which, especially in the beginning, is comparable to a continuous supply in the right lateral position. HENDERSON observed that the gastric emptying time for a child decreases gradually; this follows in the same line of thought (84).

6. Effect of the absorption of fluids from the contrast column in the distal ileum

To obtain roentgenograms of the small intestine suitable for interpretation, it will appear that it is exceedingly important that a specific fluid concentration be maintained for the contrast medium. In the jejunum some dilution will generally occur or flocculation will develop when a contrast medium of lower stability is used. In the distal ileum and especially in the colon, absorption of fluid from the contrast suspension will again increase the viscosity and specific gravity. Therefore in the distal ileum, intense white contrast areas can develop with only a few patterns of the mucosal folds. For prolonged periods in the colon, this fluid withdrawal can even lead to the formation of barium stones.

7. Obstructions in the small intestine

When there are obstructions in the small intestine, the contents of the loops above the stenosis will increase without any further fluid being added orally owing to the addition of secretion and exudation products from the intestinal wall. This results in an increasing dilution usually accompanied by flocculation of the contrast medium in the loops above the stenosis and not a dehydration as generally feared in literature. This has been demonstrated not only in hundreds of patients but also with animals (143, 155). In all literature, not one single publication can be found reporting on experiments with animals or patients whereby thickening of the contrast fluid in the loops above the obstruction in the small intestine was found. As a result of the increased tone, the peristaltic waves are initially enhanced; if the stenosis lasts somewhat longer, peristalsis decreases gradually.

SLOAN et al. (196) in a fine series of experiments with 60 dogs, showed that above the stenosis fluid increase in loops of greater width will develop within several hours and that the radiologist can only suspect a diagnosis of ileus when gas is also seen in these loops. This gas consists of 68 per cent swallowed air, 12 per cent gas caused by bacteria and 20 per cent gas exchanged from the blood via the intestinal wall.

During the same experiments, it appeared that the length of the intestinal segments above the stenosis increases gradually with time and that the viscosity of the contrast fluid decreases. It was found that several hours after the obstruction had been placed in well-hydrated dogs, the radiological diagnosis 'ileus' could be made sooner than for dehydrated dogs. In a later stage, significant differences between these 2 groups could no longer be seen. About 1960, an attempt was made to use water soluble contrast media containing iodine to localize the obstruction radiologically in what was assumed to be a safer way. In the following chapter, this will be discussed in more detail.

Possibly as time passes we shall discover that not all facets of the physiology of the small intestine which are important to the follow-through examination have been discussed, but it should now be clear that there are a number of fundamental factors with a pronounced influence on the length of the examination. These factors also help to determine the quality of the intestinal mucosal patterns on the röntgenological films; this will be discussed in the following chapter.

V
THE CONTRAST MEDIUM

General considerations

As we have seen in Chapter II, during the second world war barium was the generally accepted contrast medium for examination of the small intestine. The 40-year-old custom of mixing nutrients with the contrast medium was abandoned since this appeared to be the main reason that good mucosal patterns could not be obtained. The importance of good reproduction of anatomical detail had become considerable since the morphological examination of the small intestine had replaced the functional examination. The omission of nutrients however did not improve the characteristics of the contrast medium such that it could now be regarded as ideal and was considered satisfactory by everyone. It had been recognized that a good contrast medium suited for examination of the digestive tract must satisfy many requirements, namely (224):

1. sedimentation may not occur after prolonged standing,
2. must mix easily with all secretion and digestive products found in the stomach and the small intestine without the development of flocculation and segmentation. The contrast medium must therefore also be insensitive to pH changes,
3. must adhere readily,
4. the viscosity may vary between that of water and that of cream but no more. In order to prevent the formation of stones due to fluid absorption in the colon and the distal ileum, a specific maximum viscosity may not be exceeded,
5. barium content must be high enough for good contrast,
6. must have a homogeneous structure,
7. must have a pleasant taste,
8. must be non-toxic,
9. must be inexpensive and easy to prepare without clumping or formation of foam. Later these characteristics were expanded to include:
10. must stimulate peristalsis.

Obviously it is not easy, if at all possible, to find a contrast medium which satisfies all of these requirements. Several of these factors will be discussed separately in more detail.

1. Sedimentation of the contrast medium

A well-known characteristic of barium powder is that it precipitates quickly in aqueous solutions, as does bismuth. In 1931 HOLZKNECHT wrote in his handbook (90) that the colon mixture must be stirred until just before use. In the same book, JOZEF PALUGUAY wrote that colloidal barium suspensions were on the market which gave a better reproduction of relief and which settled less quickly. He did not see the usefulness of these new media however because the same could be achieved by first boiling and then cooling the barium suspension.

The problem of sedimentation had already been studied extensively in 1947 by the pharmacologist BRAECKMAN (22). He suggested that the formation of clumps of barium particles can be separated into an orthokinetic and perikinetic coagulation. The former pertains to the larger particles and is caused by gravitation, the latter applies to the smaller particles and is caused by Brownian movement. Although an increase in the viscosity of the solution will cause a decrease in both types of clumping, perikinetic coagulation is more effectively combatted by adding an electrolyte or peptizing agent to the contrast suspension. In addition, there is of course less coagulation when the particles are smaller; it is also important that the particles be of equal size, otherwise the larger will act as nidus (BROWN, 24).

Barium sulfate particles in water have a slight negative charge due to the OH groups on their surface. The agglomeration of these particles is decreased by increasing their negative charge. BROWN achieved this by adding a small amount of an electrolyte with many hydroxyl groups, such as sodium carboxymethylcellulose. BRAECKMAN obtained the best results in his experiments with a mixture of 7.5 per cent arabic gum and 0.01 N. sodium citrate. On a graph, he showed the differences between the rate of sedimentation of a mixture of $BaSO_4$ and 0.01 N. sodium citrate and the rate of sedimentation of the same mixture with 7.5 per cent arabic gum added (fig. 2). If too much hydrophilic colloid is

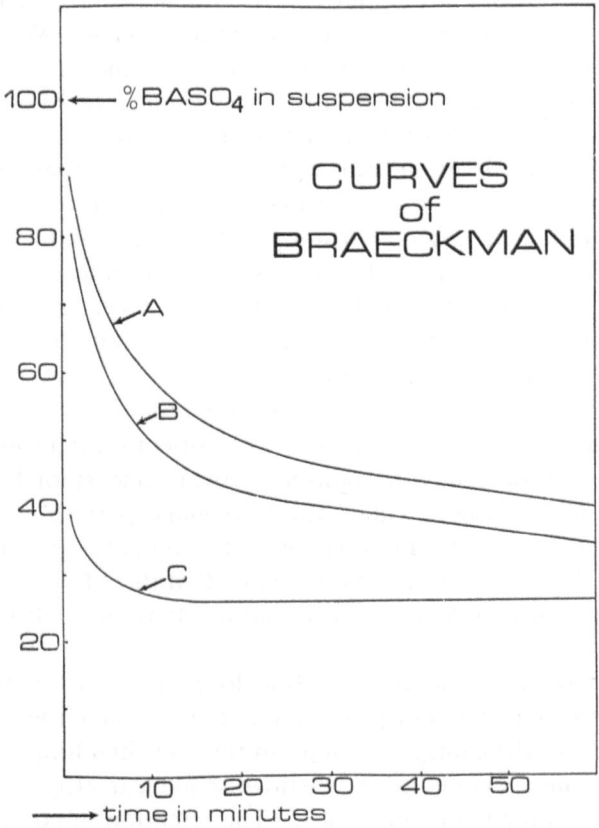

Fig. 2
Difference in rate of sedimentation of following mixtures:
A: $BaSO_4$ + 0.01 N. citr. Na + 7.5% gum. arab.
B: $BaSO_4$ + 7.5% gum. arab.
C: $BaSO_4$ + 0.01 N. citr. Na

added, then the negative charge will become too high and clumping will again occur as a result of the strong mutual repulsion. During this phenomenon, called 'super settling', a barium mass develops which is so hard and compact that it can no longer be dissolved. A suspension with such a high negative charge has the advantage of being almost insensitive to pH changes in the digestive tract. Therefore mucus and other substances found in the digestive tract will not cause flocculation. Since in any event 'super settling' must be avoided, some tendency toward flocculation is unfortunately necessary. The rate of sedimentation of many barium sulfate preparations now on the market is so low that this factor no longer plays a role in the examination of patients. The stomach and the intestine are in sufficient continuous motion to prevent pure sedimentation. LETTERS and GAUL (122) had already reached this conclusion in 1951.

2. Flocculation of the contrast fluid

A phenomenon which perhaps appears quite similar to sedimentation but must definitely be differentiated from it is the flocculation of barium particles in the contrast suspension when it comes into contact with specific substances found in the digestive tract, such as hydrochloric acid, gall and mucin. Mucin is coated with colloidal protein polymers which are usually amphoteric; it is therefore positive in acidic and negative in basic surroundings. Under normal circumstances therefore a massive clumping with the negatively charged barium particles will occur in the stomach. We observe this phenomenon as flocculation. It had already been reported in 1931 by BERG and in 1932 by FRICK (61). KNOEFEL et al. (106) demonstrated that a 10 per cent solution of barium sulfate flocculates 10 times as fast in gastric juice as in water. An increase in the amount of gastric juice causes a further increase in the rate of flocculation until a specific limiting value has been reached, apparently when all the mucoprotein has combined. Sedimentation appears to be mainly a physical process, flocculation a chemical process. A contrast medium prepared from barium powder with very tiny particles of approximately the same size, which in addition has a cream-like viscosity and contains a peptizing agent, will produce practically no sedimentation. Experience with patients has however shown that this same medium can, in spite of continuous movement, still produce pronounced flocculation when gastric acid or other juices found in the digestive tract are added. The precipitation caused by sedimentation in vitro has a homogeneous structure. Flocculation on the other hand produces a precipitation with a coarse, splotchy structure; a complete change in the viscosity of the contrast medium is even possible (fig. 4B). Also in vivo, flocculation can be recognized by the coarse, splotchy structure of the contrast medium in the intestinal lumen; this is called the 'snowflake pattern'. The finely spotted pattern usually left behind after the contrast medium has passed through the jejunum is also caused by flocculation of the barium residual. In general it can be stated that these floccules will be smaller when the contrast fluid adheres less readily to the mucosa so that less barium is left behind.

DEUCHER (41) introduced barium into isolated intestinal loops in surgical patients during the operation and induced peristalsis with an injection of prostigmin. He then made roentgenograms which showed a finely spotted distribution of the contrast medium in the intestinal loops. In addition he noted that the outline of the intestinal lumen could not be distinguished clearly (fig. 3). DEUCHER was not able to give a convincing explanation for these phenomena. The retention of contrast fluid between swollen folds which were not able to contract seemed to him the most likely explanation. He assumed that the mucosal swelling was caused by a disturbance in the blood circulation since there were no indications of an infectious process in the intestinal wall. It is clear that in fact we are confronted here with such a complete flocculation of the contrast fluid that there is no barium left in the suspension at all. The difference between the specific gravity of the suspension fluid and that of the tissue of the intestinal wall has therefore become so small that the outline of the intestinal lumen can no longer be seen.

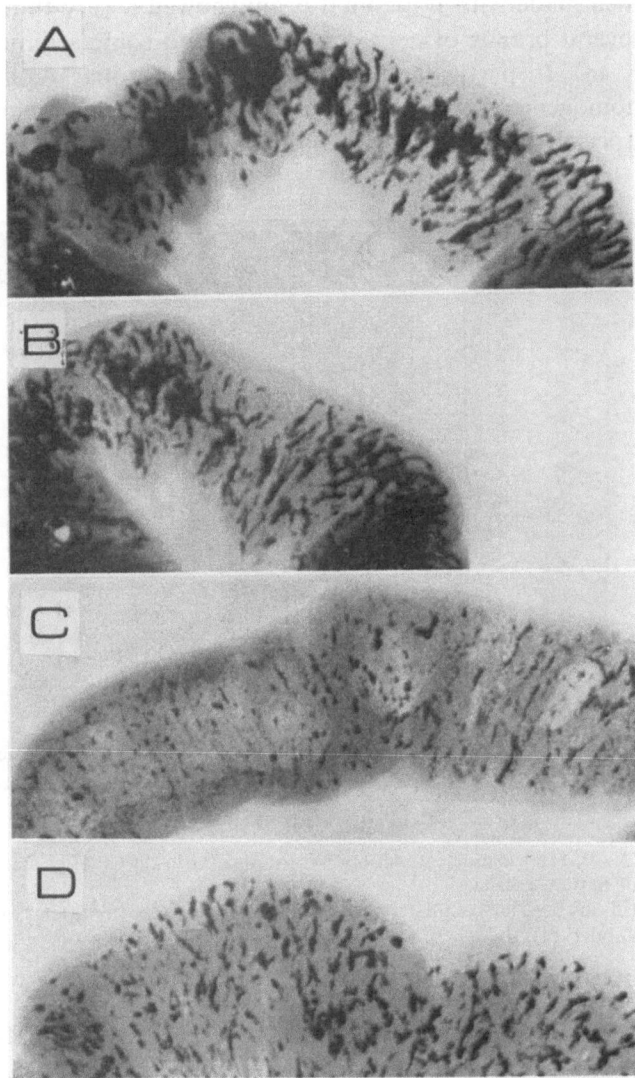

Fig. 3
Contrast fluid in isolated intestinal loop during surgery. There
is practically no barium left in suspension. Peristalsis induced
by injection of Prostigmin.
A, B: beginning of clump formation. C, D: flocculation (snowflake pattern). (DEUCHER 1949)

In my opinion, DEUCHER showed quite clearly with this experiment that no further morphological
information can be obtained once flocculation has occurred. Many radiologists have found that a
small dose of contrast medium causes more flocculation than a large dose. It has long been known
that flocculation occurs in the foremost part of the contrast column, which disappears as soon as more
contrast medium is administered (164). PATTERSON even saw flocculation develop with the exceedingly
stable Raybar which he introduced directly into the duodenum. For the patients he examined in this
way however he only used 40 ml of this contrast medium (160).

We studied the occurrence of sedimentation and flocculation by means of several experiments in vitro. Five barium suspensions of various brands were placed in test tubes, agitated and then set aside for 30 minutes. The x-ray then made with horizontal beam showed a very thin and unimportant liquid film on the surface of several brands of contrast medium and some sediment at the bottom of the test tube for others (fig. 4A). In particular the structure of Microbar AZL as well as Micropaque appears to remain very homogeneous. It is therefore obvious that the annoying effect of sedimentation no longer plays a role, especially in vivo, since then the contrast fluid is also in continuous motion.

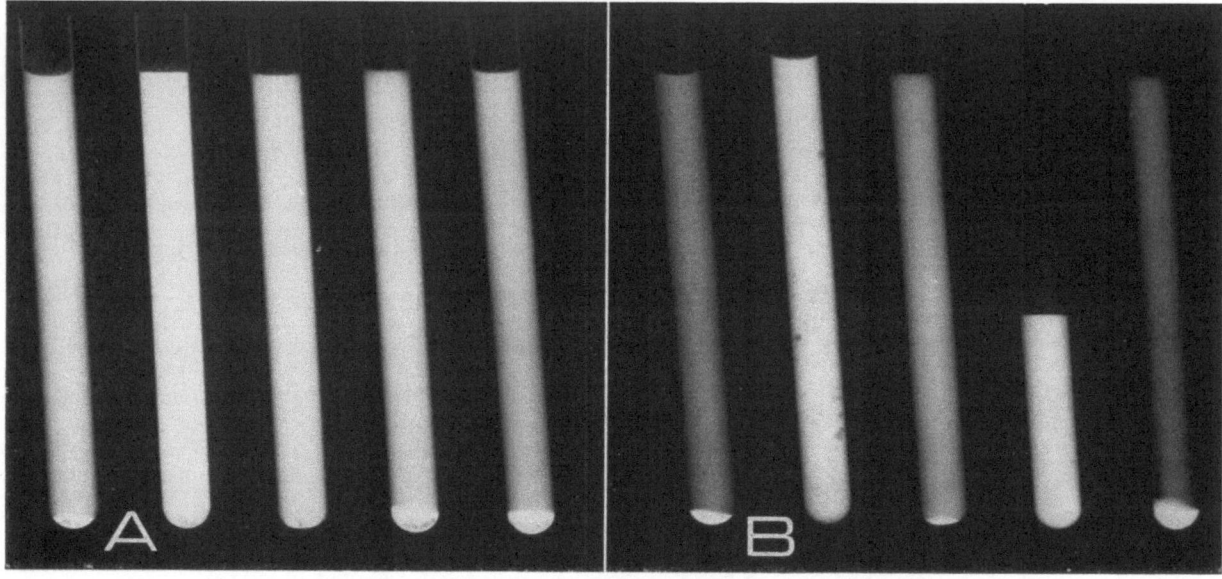

Fig. 4
A: Mixobar (1), Microbar AZL (2), Micropaque (3), Alubar W. (4) and Bario-dif (5) after standing for 30 min. Only slight sedimentation of barium particles.
B: 15 ml of the same contrast fluids used in (A) mixed with 5 ml 1/10 N. HCl. x-ray after 30 min. Microbar AZL (2) shows flocculation; for Alubar 'Wander' (4), there is practically no barium left in suspension.

The test was repeated by mixing 15 ml of the same contrast media with 5 ml 0.1 N. HCl. A contrast-acid ratio is then created which can occur under physiological circumstances. The films made after 30 min. (fig. 4B) show that the structure of Microbar AZL is definitely no longer homogeneous (flocculation). The contrast medium has acquired a gelatinous to pudding-like consistency and only after energetic shaking can it be removed from the test tube. Micropaque appeared to be insensitive to the addition of the acid while Alubar flocculated completely. This is sufficient to demonstrate that Microbar AZL is not a suitable contrast medium for either the gastric examination nor therefore the conventional method of examination of the small intestine. After mixing with hydrochloric acid, this medium does display the best adhesion on the wall of the test tube; this is probably due to the great increase in viscosity. Without the acid, the other brands adhere more readily than Microbar AZL, probably again owing to the greater viscosity of these contrast media. Although most brands of contrast medium on the market can withstand basic substances better than acidic, tests have shown that their characteristics can change greatly under influence of intestinal juice (56, 225). It is therefore clear that in vivo barium suspensions can loose their most valuable characteristics completely.

It was exceedingly difficult for the chemical industry to produce a contrast medium which retains its stability in both acidic and basic surroundings. Fig. 4B shows that not yet every manufacturer has been successful in this respect.

The fact that the factors responsible for flocculation of the contrast medium were not recognized is certainly the most important reason for the slow development of the radiological differential diagnosis of diseases of the small intestine. GOLDEN assumed that the flocculation and subsequent disintegration into segment clumps of the contrast column resulted from a disturbed motor function of the small intestine, which is a dominant symptom of sprue and is caused by abnormalities in the intramural nervous system of the intestinal wall (74). BOUSLOG (21) agreed with GOLDEN's interpretation because the nervous system in the intestinal wall of babies only a few months old is still underdeveloped and during the examination of the small intestine of these babies, he observed only that the contrast fluid flocculates and finally disintegrates into segment clumps. CAFFEY supported the assumption of a disordered motor function by reporting that passage through the small intestine lasted 5 to 6 hours for new-born children. In addition some radiologists, including GOLDEN, FRIEDMAN (59) and GOIN (71) had found that fear and emotions could cause sudden flocculation of the barium suspension, a phenomenon which is said to have also been observed in animals.

Many other radiologists, even including REYNOLDS et al. (178) in 1940, proved convincingly that flocculation of the contrast fluid can at least be caused by factors other than the above-mentioned, such as gastric acid, hypertonic solutions, proteins and fats. The authority of GOLDEN was however so great that his neurogenic theory was still generally accepted.

Not until 1949 were many converted by the publication of FRAZER, FRENCH and THOMPSON (56), who used an extensive series of tests to show that flocculation of the barium suspension in the small intestine of completely normal individuals can be caused by many factors. To avoid the influence of gastric acid, the contrast medium as well as the substances to be tested were administered through a tube directly into the duodenum. They observed flocculation followed by segmentation after adding: hypertonic solutions, acetic acid, lactic acid, fatty acids, olive oil, unsaturated fatty acids (sprue patients) and gastric mucus. Gall only caused flocculation in acidic surroundings, not for a pH greater than 6.4. To rebut GOLDEN's theory in a spectacular manner, they demonstrated that the barium suspension also flocculated in the intestines of a deceased person where a disordered motor function such as GOLDEN supposed cannot possibly exist. Furthermore it appeared that flocculation followed by segmentation developed in persons who had consumed a meal rich in fats the evening before the examination.

In the same year, ZIMMER (224) compared the characteristics of Alubar, which he considered to be a superior contrast medium, with those of an ordinary barium sulfate suspension and two commercial products by adding artificial gastric juice with a pH of 1.8–2 and artificial intestinal juice with a pH of 8.2–8.4. The roentgenograms made show varying degrees of structural change for at least 2 of the 4 contrast fluids (figs. 5B and 5C) which are highly similar to the changes noted for Microbar AZL during our experiments (fig. 4B). The rate of flocculation under the influence of gastric and intestinal juices was also measured for these 4 contrast fluids; the resulting values were plotted on a graph (fig. 5A). He then studied the homogeneity and the adhesion for these suspensions. Alubar appeared to be better than the ordinary $BaSO_4$ in all respects. In his conclusion he writes that the use of a pure $BaSO_4$ suspension will often lead to the unjustified diagnosis of sprue.

One year later, ARDRAN, FRENCH and MUCKLOW (8) also proved that a colloidal barium suspension does not flocculate in children with coeliac disease, but that a normal barium suspension does. After these publications many others of similar intent followed, but there are still radiologists who have remained more or less loyal to GOLDEN's theory of disordered motor function. In 1959, GOLDEN himself seemed to have similar difficulties in abandoning his original line of thought when he wrote:

'Flocculation is undoubtedly caused by the contents of the intestine and has been attributed to mucus. In as much as mucus is always present the question arises as to whether this effect is related to the quantity or to some unknown quality of the mucus. Flocculation may occur as a result of emotional disturbances. It may appear and disappear in an individual during a period of an hour or two for no obvious reason' (73).

Meanwhile, he prefers barium suspensions which do not flocculate but does not see any advantage in all kinds of special examination techniques.

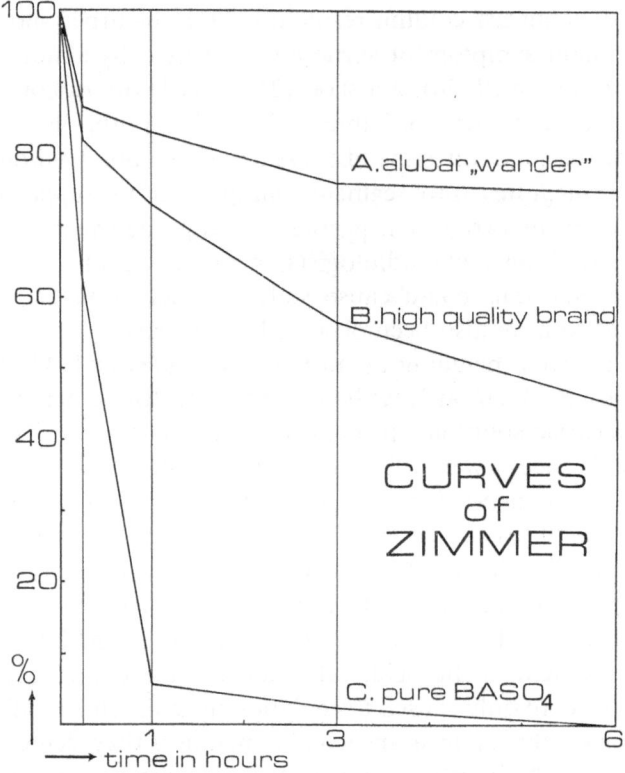

Fig. 5

A: Sedimentation curves of ZIMMER (1949). Difference between Alubar 'Wander', a high quality brand and a barium suspension without additives.

He still administers 240 ml contrast medium orally and if necessary, takes spot films. Since GIANTURCO's article in 1953, he uses the 'high voltage' technique because with a low voltage only marginal information is obtained (fig. 6).

At a congress in 1960, in reference to a demonstration of the radiologic examination of the small intestine where a tumor was not localized, GOLDEN clearly indicated that his opinions had changed in the meantime by stating: 'It would seem that a tumor such as this should easily be detected by a small intestine study (barium follow-through). The segmentation was so great and the distribution so uneven that the tumor could not be demonstrated. It seems possible that this might have been demonstrated by a small bowel enema'.

3. Segmentation of the contrast column

Although the disintegration of the contrast column into segment clumps is usually observed together with flocculation, a separate discussion of this phenomenon is justified for several reasons.

The segmentation picture was known long before that of flocculation. The reason is that flocculation is only obtained when the patient receives a reasonably homogeneous suspension of relatively small

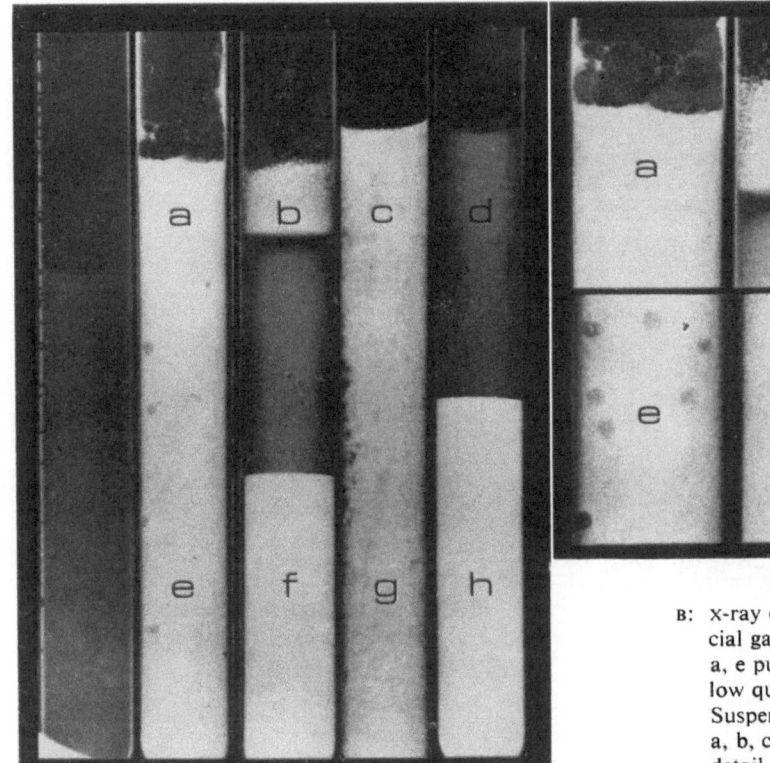

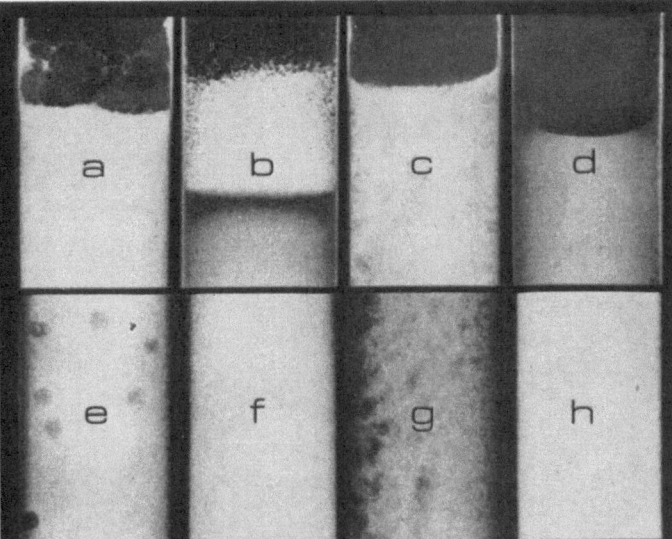

B: x-ray of 4 barium sulfate suspensions to which artificial gastric juice (pH 1.8–2) is added.
a, e pure barium sulfate; b, f high quality brand; c, g low quality brand; d, h Alubar 'Wander';
Suspensions a, e and c, g show flocculation.
a, b, c, d: detail exposures of fluid surface; e, f. g, h: detail exposures below fluid surface.

Fig. 5

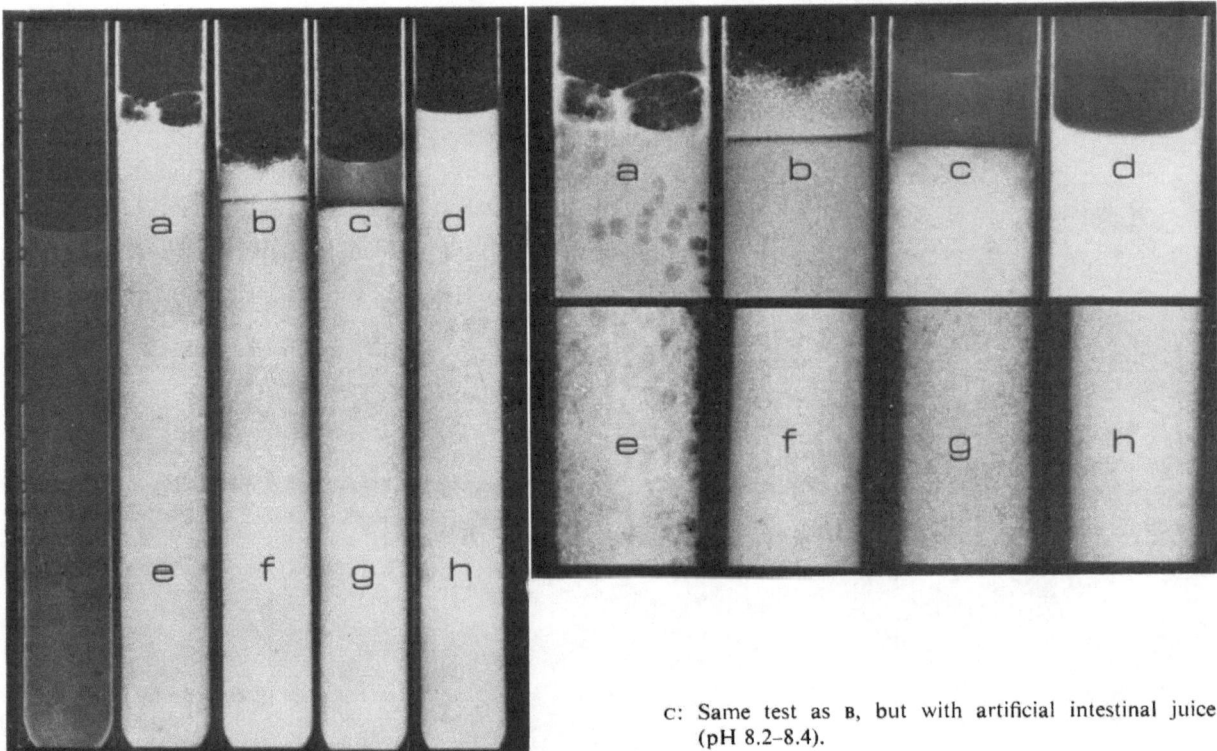

C: Same test as B, but with artificial intestinal juice (pH 8.2–8.4).

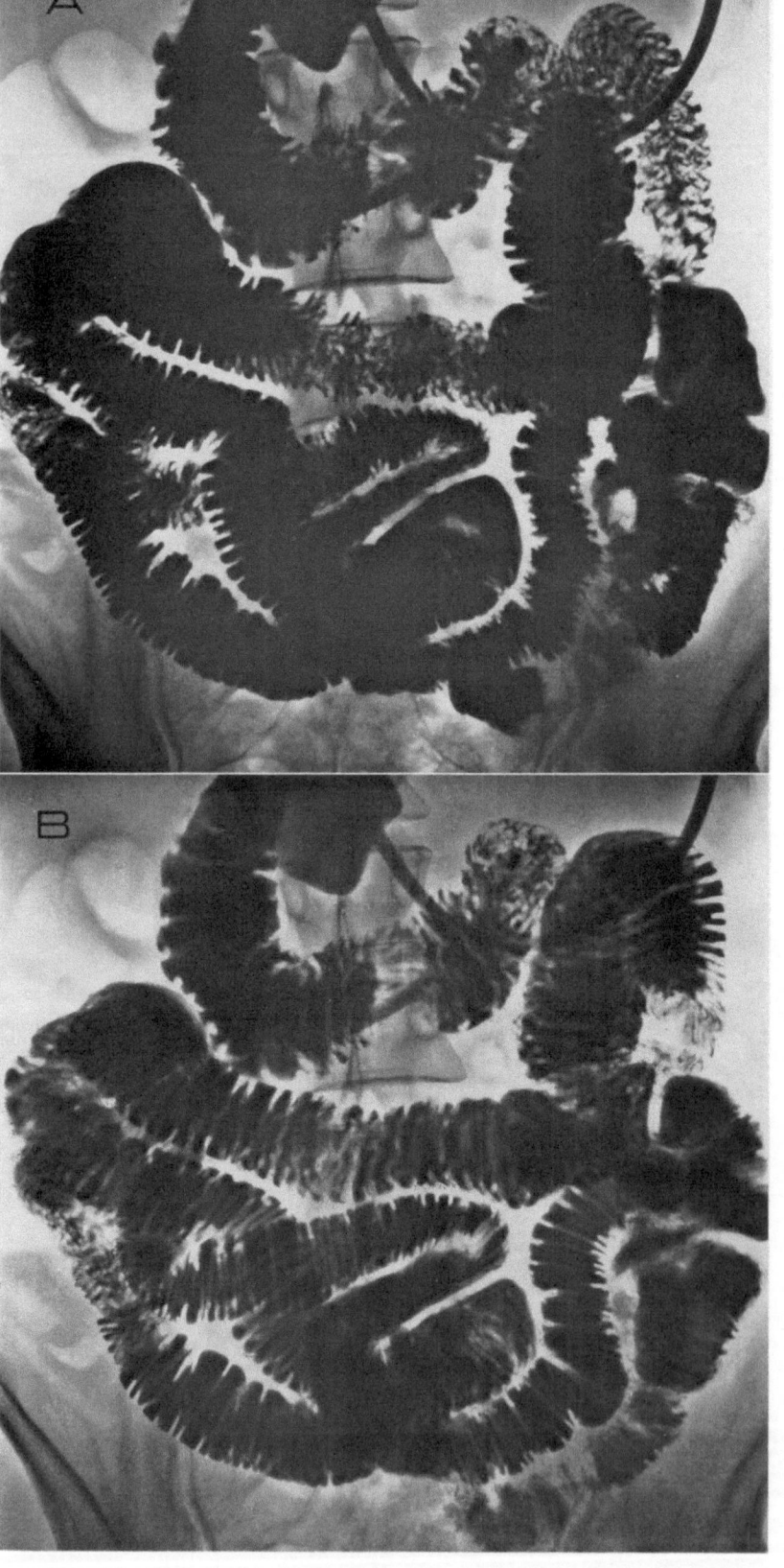

Fig. 6
Decrease of contrast by increasing
voltage. A: 80 kV. B: 120 kV.
Film density equal for both exposures.

particles. When it was still customary to mix nutrients through the contrast medium, this requirement was certainly not satisfied. As mentioned previously, owing to the withdrawal of fluids from the contrast column, segmentation in the colon is a physiological phenomenon; this is also the case in the ileum when transit is very slow. In the fluid-rich duodenum and jejunum such massive flocculation can occur that this can result in increasingly large conglomerates and finally segment clumps. In the thirties, this phenomenon was frequently seen in the duodenum and jejunum of infants; a reasonable explanation was unknown (21). Autopsy material had shown that mucosal folds were definitely present; the fact that HENDERSON had indeed observed these folds on röntgenological films when the stomach emptied rapidly also could not be explained (84).

In 1934, SNELL and CAMP described the segmentation of the contrast column in sprue. They saw clumping of the barium and disappearance of the fold relief. They are to be respected for the fact that even then they believed that this was not a specific symptom but that the same could be observed for other 'diffuse infections'. In 1939 KANTOR (102) described the 'moulage sign' which can be seen in the duodenum or jejunum, where the rigid barium column resembles a wax mold without fold relief. He only saw this picture in highly advanced cases of sprue and therefore he thought that in these cases the fold relief was greatly flattened or absent all together. In fact there will probably always be a heavy and early occurrence of clumping of the barium suspension in such cases. When the roentgenograms are overexposed, then a grainy structure of the barium column is to be expected (fig. 34B); in a case of pure mucosal atrophy, without signs of malabsorption this structure must be homogeneous. KANTOR's conclusion that the moulage sign could be considered an indication of the severity of the sprue often might still be correct, in spite of the opinion of SNELL and CAMP; however this picture has absolutely nothing to do with the condition of the mucous membrane.

In 1961 MARSHAK (132) was of the opinion that the moulage sign could be the result of hypersecretion and segmentation but in the same article he does mention his surprise that he also saw string sign-like configurations and coarse mucosal folds, which do not seem to agree with the normal autopsy findings. The quality of the published roentgenograms is however poor and they are so dominated by pictures distorted by flocculation and segmentation that this incongruity between radiological and autopsy findings is not strange. Fig. 31B and fig. 61 show that the flocculation and segment formation of the barium suspension lead to an apparent flattening and coarsening of the mucosal folds. Comparison of fig. 33 with fig. 34 shows that patterns are even possible which do not resemble the actual situation in the least.

From the above it must be concluded that a radiological examination of the small intestine should be terminated when the contrast fluid shows clear signs of disintegration and is apparently no longer able to provide real images of the intestinal mucosa. It would be ideal if a contrast medium was available which is highly stable, moderately viscous and adheres readily. In order to prevent the annoying effect of dehydration and thickening of the barium column in the distal ileum during slow transit, it is also desirable that the contrast medium be protected against unlimited fluid withdrawal. Of the numerous attempts undertaken to improve the characteristics of the contrast media, only the most important shall be discussed.

4. Additives to the contrast medium for the purpose of improving stability and adhesion

Many radiologists have tried this method to increase the adhesion of the contrast medium to the mucous membrane of the digestive tract. An improvement in adhesion is usually also accompanied by a decrease in the sedimentation and flocculation tendencies of the contrast medium; therefore an attempt aimed specifically at the latter cannot easily be distinguished from the former. Due to the importance of double-contrast exposures for the colon examination, good adhesion is even more important for this examination than for an examination of the small intestine, while the reverse holds for sedimentation and flocculation. Adhesion of the barium meal to the intestinal mucosa could be increased by adding tannin since this substance causes precipitation of proteins on the surface cellular layers and decreases the mucin secretion.

For a long time, tannin was used for the colon examination in concentrations of 0.3 to 3 per cent in the cleansing enema and in the contrast medium. Since it has become known that tannin is absorbed by the mucous membrane (107) and 8 fatal cases resulting from necrosis of the liver have been described, use of this substance has been forbidden in America (6). Some do not agree with this decision since they believe that in these cases, the possibility of overdosage exists (95). Tannin is found in tea and, it is said, in red wine. It is not only hepatotoxic but is also believed to be carcinogenic. When perforations occur and the barium mixture containing tannin enters the abdominal cavity, a serious chemical peritonitis develops. To avoid lethal termination acute surgical intervention and cleaning of the abdominal cavity is absolutely necessary.

As far as we know, tannin has never played a role of any importance in the examination of the small intestine although the influence of a cup of strong tea consumed the evening before the examination has never been studied.

In 1938 WOOLDMAN (216) reported that the addition of colloidal aluminum hydroxyde to the contrast medium produced good results. This substance is slightly astringent, does not irritate and is amphoteric. He had noticed during operations and in autopsy material that a contrast medium containing this substance adheres quite readily to the mucosa.

In 1953, SHUFFLEBARGER et al. (193) tried to improve adhesion to the mucous membrane by decreasing the secretion of the intestinal wall in animals and later also patients. They injected histamine and atropine but were not successful. They did note that the best results were obtained in patients with hypotonic, ptotic stomachs.

ALEXANDER (5) believed that adhesion would be improved if the barium suspension mixed easily with the mucus; he therefore added 1 per cent mucin. He reported improvement for the examination of the small intestine and the colon, but not for the esophageal and gastric examinations.

EMBRING and MATTSSON (45) added a wetting agent (tweens, sodium lauryl sulfate and saponins) to enhance the mixing of 2 different water phases, but they were not very enthusiastic about their results.

Many radiologists (24, 45, 105, 163 and others) added carboxymethyl cellulose or its sodium salt to the barium suspension and in general reported good results with this combination. The sodium CMC does cause an increase in viscosity but does not dissolve in gastric juice and does not appear to adhere as readily as the CMC in a 0.5 per cent concentration. Both substances are highly hydrophilic and therefore accelerate transit.

Both the binding of water and the acceleration of transit protect the barium suspension against excessive fluid withdrawal in the ileum. A slight disadvantage of the contrast media containing hydrophilic colloids to restrict dehydration in the ileum is that they cannot be used to diagnose a disaccharidase deficiency (112). Micropaque therefore does not contain these colloids; however for prolonged transit times there is the disadvantage of pronounced dehydration in the distal ileum as a result of fluid withdrawal. Other substances which have occasionally been used to improve the adhesion of the contrast medium are tragacanth and arabic gum (2, 84). The results described vary widely; this may be a result of the various dosages used. HENDERSON did not see any improvements when 10 ml 2 per cent arabic gum was added, an observation which we can confirm. We have found that the addition of 10 volume per cent of the total amount of the contrast medium, thus a considerably higher dosage, does produce satisfactory results. This suspension however is rather viscous and only becomes thinner and more liquid in patients with sufficient gastric acid. This decrease in viscosity is not accompanied by flocculation at all; in this case the gastric acid is apparently bound chemically. This chemical combining of the gastric acid must be regarded as specifically preventing flocculation; substances which bind mucin have the same effect. In addition to the above-mentioned substances, many others have been tested; as a result it has been demonstrated clearly that no single additive has been found which is ideal. Some of these substances are: buttermilk, olive oil, sodium oleate, fecal fat from sprue patients, diverse carbohydrates, lactic acid, citric acid, gelatin, agar and pectin.

It is unfortunate that only 4 years ago EMBRING and MATTSSON (45) again propagated a more physiological contrast medium containing protein, fat and carbohydrates. Hopefully further study of the literature and of their own roentgenograms has convinced them to abandon these attempts.

5. Relationship between viscosity, particle size and adhesion of the barium suspension

Although the adhesive capacity of a suspension can be increased by adding several substances, a minimum viscosity is also a necessary requirement. An increase in the viscosity however has the disadvantage of retarding the rate of transit through the pylorus and small intestine. An additional difficulty is that when the viscosity of the contrast medium is too high, the adhesive layer left behind can become annoyingly thick (fig. 7). The correct (creamy) viscosity for the suspension however does not guarantee that adhesion will be good.

Some radiologists have tried to obtain a clearly visible adhesive layer by preparing solutions with a high specific gravity and a very low viscosity. One example is Brown's mixture (24). He used sodium carboxymethyl cellulose, heparin and sodium dextran sulfate or sodium cellulose acetate to obtain a thin, liquid suspension containing 75 weight per cent barium. For this contrast medium BROWN reports a short transit time of only 1 to 1.5 hours, but unfortunately he does not mention the amounts administered nor other details of fundamental importance for the evaluation of the medium. EMBRING and MATTSSON (44) also obtained a thin, liquid, as well as stable barium suspension with a specific gravity of approximately 3 as follows: they added 1 g sodium citrate and 9 g Sorbitol to a paste-like mixture of 100 g $BaSO_4$ and 40 ml water; a pronounced decrease in viscosity resulted. However for filling exposures of even the relatively thin ileum a barium suspension with a specific gravity of 3 is much too high and therefore not desirable; only marginal diagnoses can be made with this medium (p. 33).

For double-contrast exposures, it is in principle a question of personal preference whether a thin liquid suspension with a high specific gravity or a thicker liquid suspension with a lower specific gravity is used; a clearly visible layer can be obtained with both.

Various radiologists, even including ADAM (2) in 1932, have shown that for a good adhesive layer in double-contrast exposures, the colloidal chemical relationships are more important than the particle size. For suspensions with a low viscosity a particle size of less than 0.4 microns can even be a disadvantage instead of an advantage. Both the specific gravity and the thickness of the adhesive layer are then insufficient for the double-contrast examination and thus all the factors for a barely visible adhesive layer are present. A striking example of this is the 50 per cent Microbar AZL which has a specific gravity of 1.32, a very low viscosity and a particle size of only 0.1 to 0.3 microns. This contrast medium therefore was not suitable for double-contrast exposures.

BROWN pointed out that for the same weight of barium, the viscosity of a suspension increases as the size of the particles decreases and that the adhesion decreases as soon as the barium content in a suspension becomes greater than 45 weight per cent. Many who have prepared barium suspensions

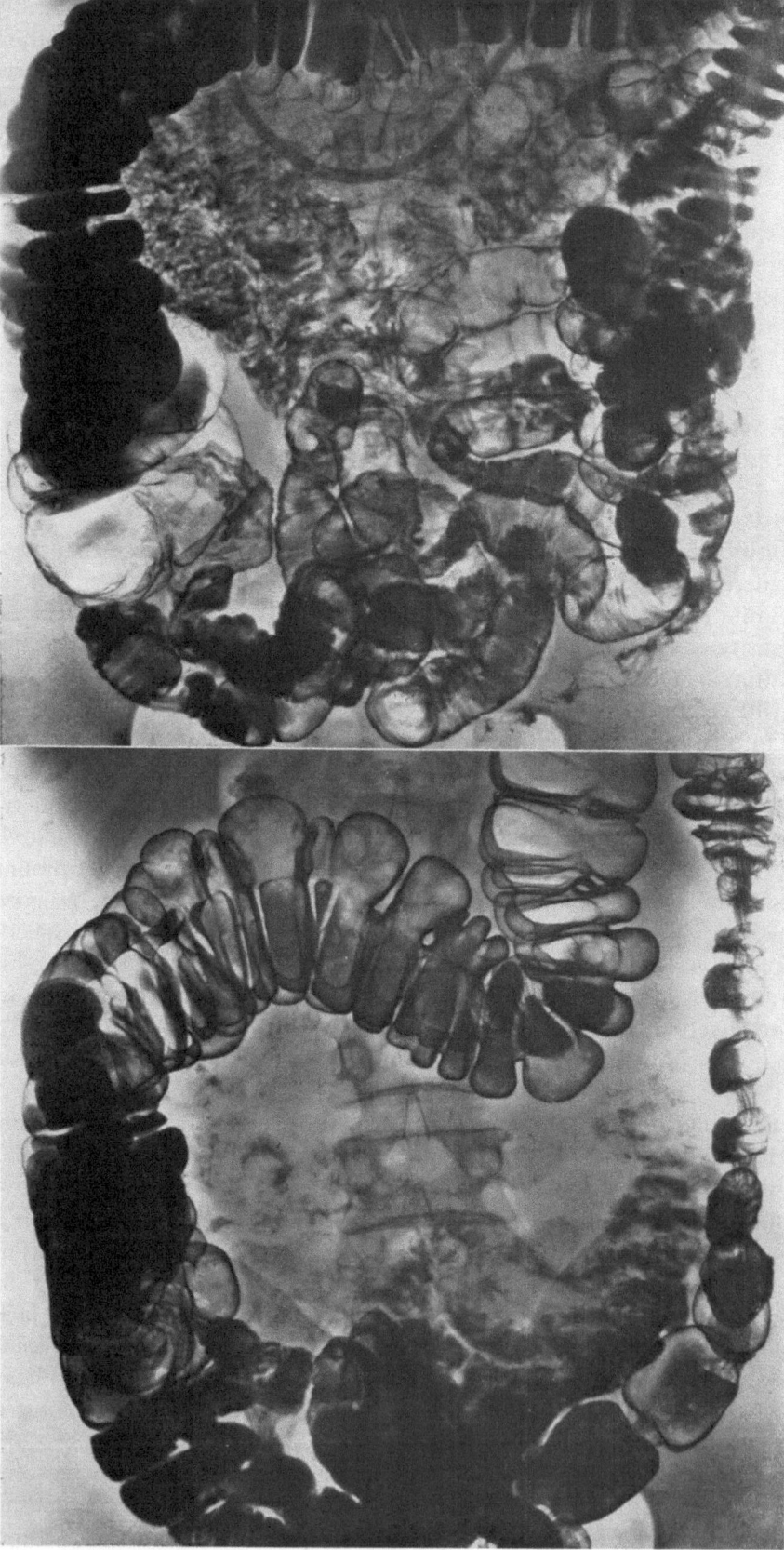

Fig. 7
Double contrast exposure of
large and small intestine. Air
injected through duodenal tube.
The s.g. of the contrast fluid is
too high (undiluted Bario-dif,
s.g. 1.45) and the adhesive layer
is too thick.

themselves for an examination of the esophageal varices will have experienced the truth of this observation.

When requested, the manufacturers of contrast media usually do not supply adequate information about the chemical composition of their product. It was found that often the data supplied were not even correct; this was also true for the particle size given.

Microscopic studies have proven that the grains were usually much larger than indicated, sometimes even significantly larger than prescribed by the American pharmacopeia (145). In addition the relative differences in the grain size of the diverse products on the market appeared to be a factor of 4 (44). SHUFFLEBARGER et al. (193) made diagrams of the grain size distribution of 6 different brands of barium sulfate and showed that most of the powders also displayed a marked lack of homogeneity. MORETON and YATES (147) compared 4 commercial preparations and obtained similar results.

6. Specific gravity of the contrast fluid

We have found that generally this exceedingly important factor has not received sufficient attention and often barium suspensions are used with a specific gravity which is much too high. The choice of the barium content for a suspension is apparently influenced by the spectacular sight of snow-white intestinal loops, preferably against the background blackening of a normally exposed abdominal survey film. As long as there are no annoying effects of superposition, only small abnormalities on the contours of the intestinal loops can be seen clearly on these photographs. In addition the other organs in the abdomen will also be seen since their blackening falls in the midportion of the density curve (fig. 8, section D). Masses in the lumen of the intestine, however, will be easily missed since there is insufficient contrast difference with the intense white parts of the intestinal loops which lie in the lowermost part of the density curve (fig. 8, section A). It will be obvious that with this exposure technique, only 2 very small segments of the contours of these snow-white intestinal loops are visible. The specific gravity of the human body differs only slightly from that of water and can be set at approximately 1. The specific gravity of a concentrated barium suspension, such as undiluted liquid Micropaque, is approximately 1.75. The difference in specific gravity between this contrast fluid and the human body is approximately 0.75, thus even less than the difference in specific gravity between the human body and air which is slightly less than 1.

From this it could be concluded that air could perhaps be an ideal as well as very inexpensive contrast medium for the examination of the digestive tract. However a disadvantage of air is that its specific gravity cannot be regulated by means of dilution like the positive contrast media. In addition air is not capable of adhering to the mucosa and therefore cannot leave traces of its presence. Air is also not able to mix with mucus secretion and therefore cannot penetrate the narrow spaces which are filled with fluids. The greatest disadvantage of air however is that disturbing fluctuations caused by solitary gas bubbles are located in approximately the same section of the density curve as fluctuations of the intestinal loops filled with gas. The result is that an isolated gas bubble for instance could not be differentiated from a diverticulum of either the anterior or the posterior intestinal wall. Unhindered evaluation of the intestinal loops and the contrast fluctuations caused by diverticula and polypoid tumors can best be made when:

1. the density of these loops differs markedly from that of the (irrelevant) background and its fluctuations,
2. the contrast fluctuations caused by pathological processes of the intestinal wall fall in the steep part of the density curve and can therefore be seen as clearly as possible,

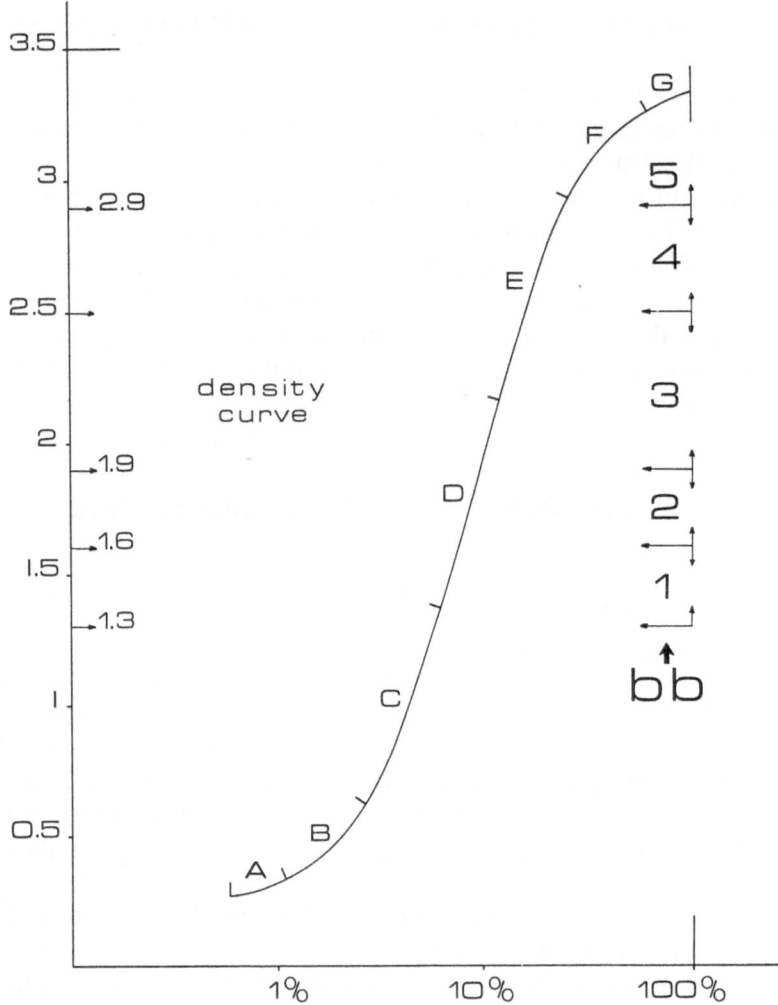

Fig. 8
Schematical representation of a film density curve. Background blackenings 1, 2, 3, 4 and 5 (figs. 8–15) are indicated on the curve.

3. the background fluctuations fall in the highest possible section of the density curve, and therefore cause the least possible disturbance.

From the above, it can be seen that theoretically the density of the intestinal loops can best fall in section C and the density for the rest of the abdomen in section G of this curve. The specific gravity of the contrast fluid should then be chosen such that small outpouchings of the intestinal lumen and narrow fistulous tracts can be seen clearly on the one hand, while on the other hand, mucosal folds and small masses, even in the lumen of wide loops, do not escape our attention. It is known that a high voltage exposure technique levels out the contrasts; this has a favourable effect on the density, of both the background and the intestinal loops filled with contrast fluid (fig. 6). A film blackening such that the background falls in section G of the curve would, however, mean a very high radiation dose for the patient.

Therefore we thought it would be useful to experiment with a phantom to determine how much the background blackening with its fluctuations can be decreased without interfering with the evaluation of the contrast differences in the intestinal loops. It also seemed worthwhile during these experiments to test contrast fluids of different specific gravity in order to determine which specific gravity (s.g.) gives maximum information.

In a 15 cm thick phantom filled with water which acted as scattering medium, we placed plastic pipes with diameters of 22 and 34 mm. The plastic pipes were filled with barium suspensions with s.g. of 1.65, 1.32 and 1.2. In each plastic pipe was a nylon thread holding wooden beads with diameters of 5, 7, 9, and 12 mm. Roentgenograms were made with a voltage of 125 kV and increasing degrees of background blackening (henceforth designated as: b.b.), numbered from 1 to 5. These 5 levels were chosen such that they adequately represented the upper half of the density curve (fig. 8). The walls of the plastic pipes could still be seen with b.b. 3; with b.b.4 they were no longer clearly visible.

The results were as follows:

I.   For the contrast medium with a s.g. of 1.65 in the 22 mm pipe, the largest bead could be seen vaguely with b.b. 2; not until b.b. 4 were all 4 beads visible in this pipe. They could be observed most clearly with b.b. 5 in the 34 mm pipe, the 3 largest beads were just visible with b.b. 5 (fig. 9).

II. For the contrast fluid with a s.g. of 1.32 in the 22 mm pipe, visibility of all 4 beads increased as the b.b. increased from 2 to 4.

Although clearer with b.b. 4, all 4 beads in the 34 mm pipe were already visible with b.b. 3; the smallest was very vague. With b.b. 2 no beads were visible in the large pipe (fig. 10).

III. For the contrast fluid with a s.g. of 1.2, the visibility of all 4 beads in both pipes increased as the b.b. increased from 1 to 3 (fig. 11).

IV. In the small pipe, the beads in the contrast fluid with a s.g. of 1.32 and a certain b.b. were as clearly visible as the beads in the contrast fluid with a s.g. of 1.2 and one b.b. lower.

V.   When the film density is even higher, the same applies for the large pipe.

The contrast fluid with a s.g. of 1.2 revealed the beads in the large pipe somewhat more clearly with b.b. 2 than the fluid with a s.g. of 1.32 with b.b. 3. This difference in visibility of the beads in the large pipe increases as the b.b. decreases to the advantage of the contrast fluid with the lowest specific gravity.

The experiment was repeated but this time the wooden beads were not located in the middle of the plastic pipes but along the wall. Fig. 12 shows the results, which are similar to those of the previous experiment. Once again it was apparent that the wooden beads are most clearly visible when the film density is high; in all cases however with the same b.b. they are more clearly visible than in the previous experiment. There is again no difference in clearness in the small pipe between a s.g. of 1.32 with a certain b.b. and a s.g. of 1.2 with one b.b. less. In the large pipe, however, as the b.b. decreases the beads were significantly clearer in the contrast fluid with the lowest specific gravity.

The results with a s.g. of 1.65 were again very disappointing, although somewhat less than in the previous experiment.

For the actual examination of the digestive tract, the results of these experiments offer the following:

1. A s.g. of 1.65 is always much too high for the contrast fluid and a b.b. in the lower half of the density curve is always too low. A combination of these 2 factors is particularly unfavourable, especially for a colon examination.
2. The combination of a relatively high b.b. (approx. 3) and a contrast fluid with a low s.g. yields the most information. When the s.g. of the contrast fluid is decreased, the b.b. can also be decreased without a loss of information. This means a lower radiation dose for the patient.
3. For the colon examination, the specific gravity of the contrast fluid must be lower than for a transit examination and the blackening of the background must be higher.
4. The loss in information due to underexposure of the x-ray films is less when a contrast fluid with a low specific gravity is used. The loss in information due to a contrast fluid with a high specific gravity can be compensated by overexposure of the x-ray film.

In order to evaluate the disturbance caused by fluctuations in the background blackening, a new

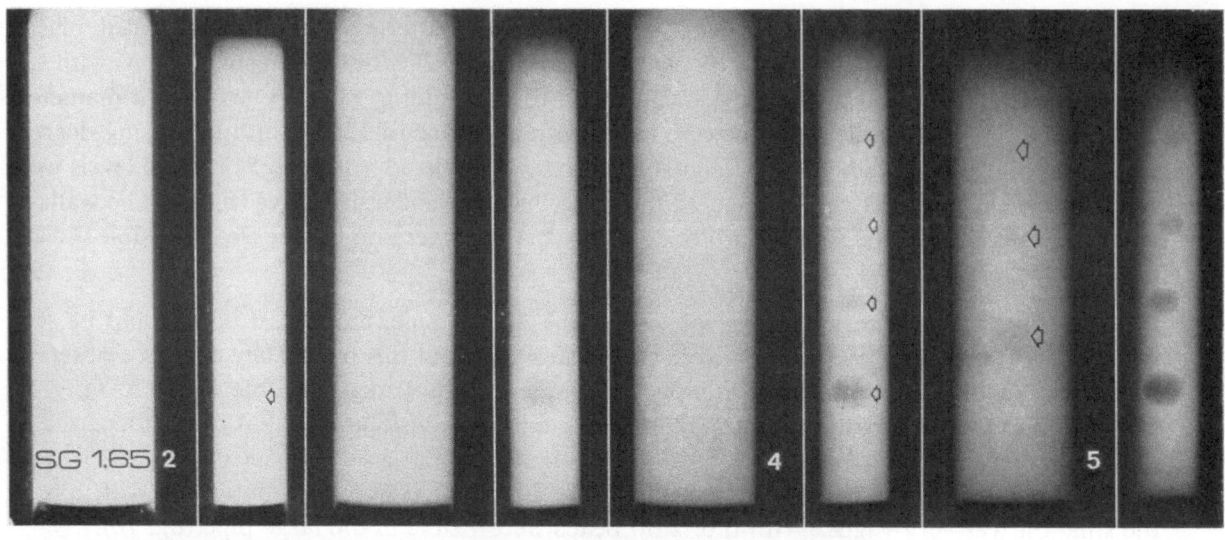

Fig. 9

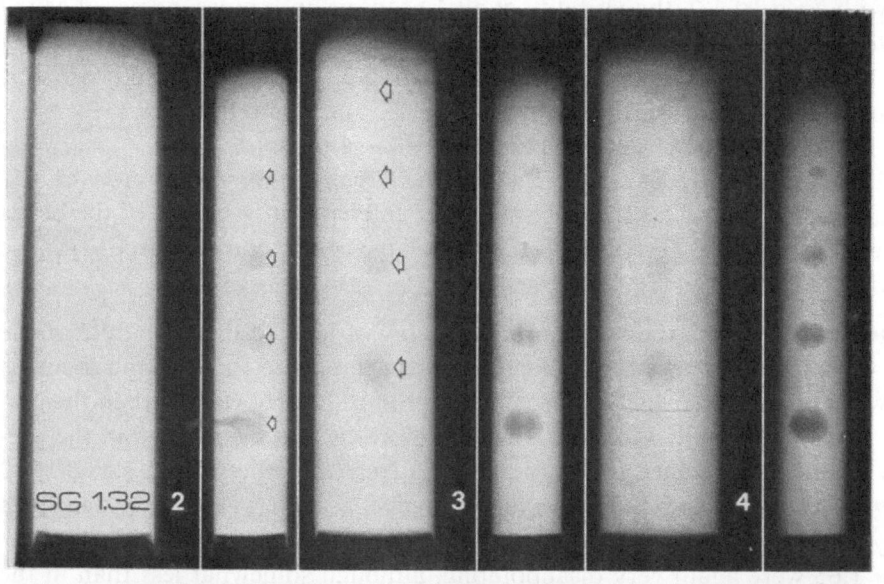

Fig. 10

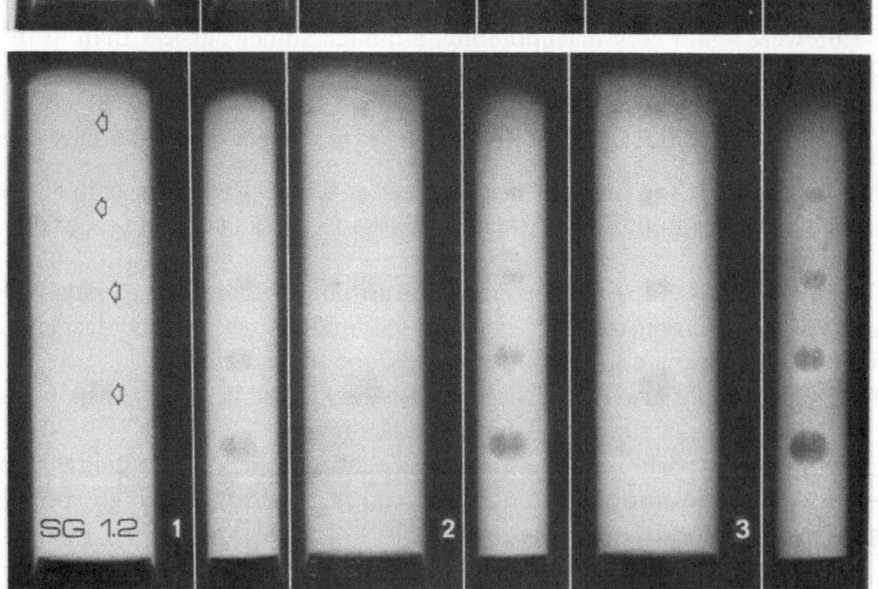

Fig. 11

Fig. 12

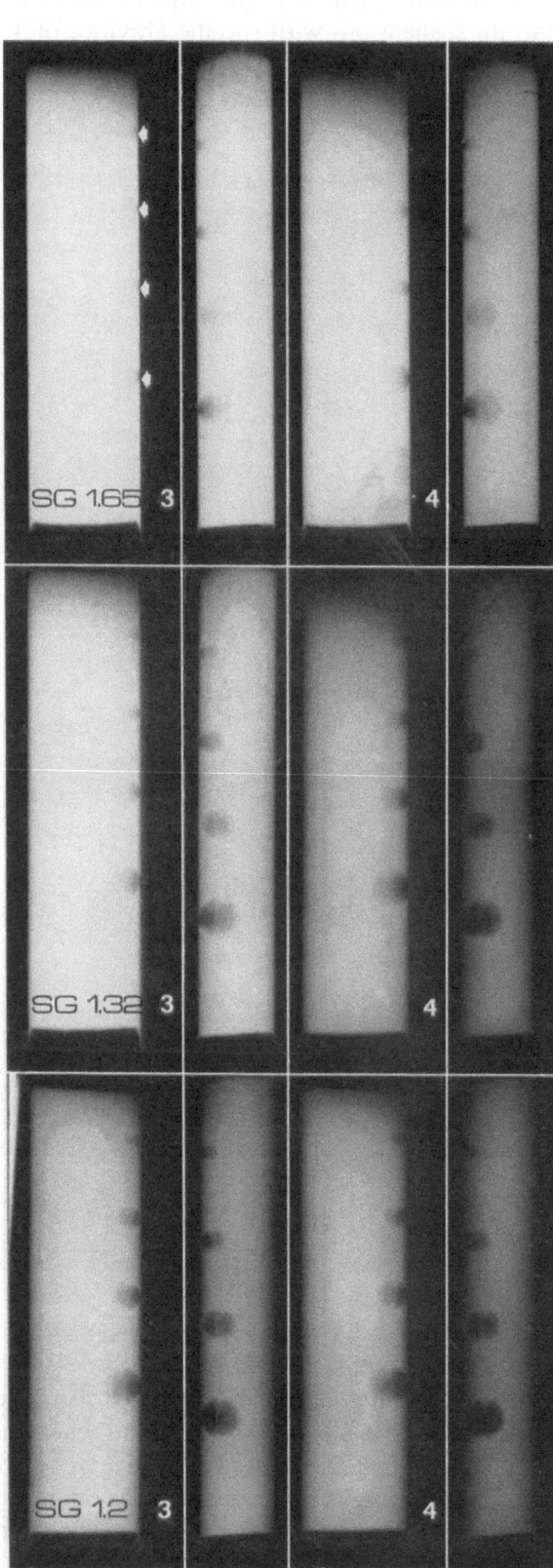

Figs. 9–14
Tests on the s.g. of the contrast fluid.The diameters of the
plastic pipes are 14, 22 and 34 mm and of the wooden beads,
5, 7, 8 and 12 mm.
The background blackening (B.b.) is shown in white numbers;
the values 1 through 5 correspond to the following values on
the density curve (fig. 8):

1 → 1.3 — 1.6	4 → 2.5 — 2.9
2 → 1.6 — 1.9	5 → > 2.9
3 → 1.9 — 2.5	

experiment was carried out. A transverse, air-filled plastic pipe 22 mm in diameter was introduced into the water phantom. This pipe crossed the 2 pipes filled with contrast fluid. This time we used barium suspensions with specific gravities of 1.32 and 1.16, and once again exposures with varying b.b. were made.

The results were as follows (fig. 13):

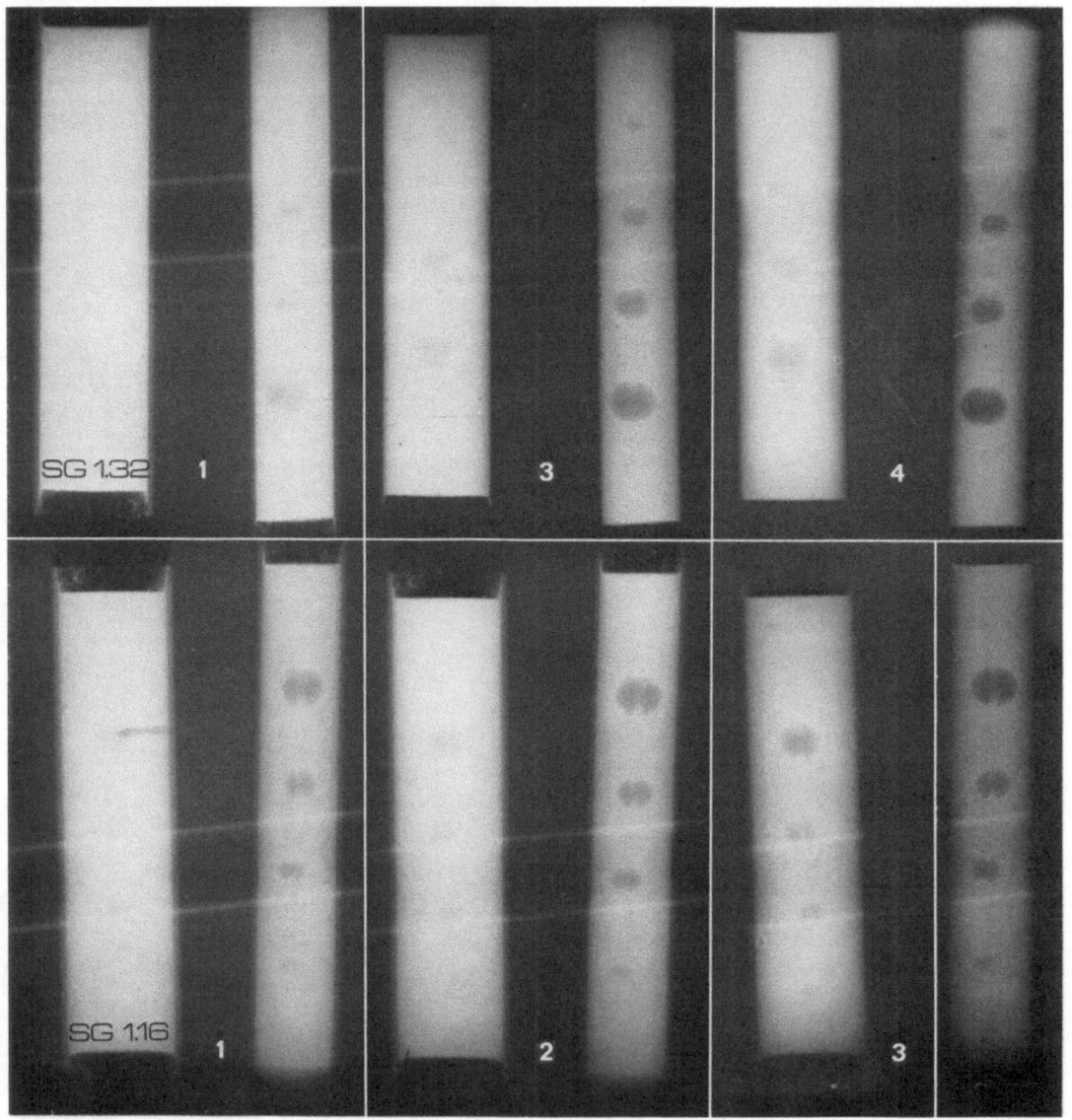

Fig. 13

1. The disturbing influence of the contrast fluctuations caused by the lumen and the wall of the air pipe is the least for the background when the density is high (sections F and G) and for the pipes filled with contrast fluid, when the density is low (sections A and B).
2. The disturbing positive and negative influences of the air pipe are greater for the background as the density decreases and for the contrast column as the specific gravity of the barium suspension decreases.

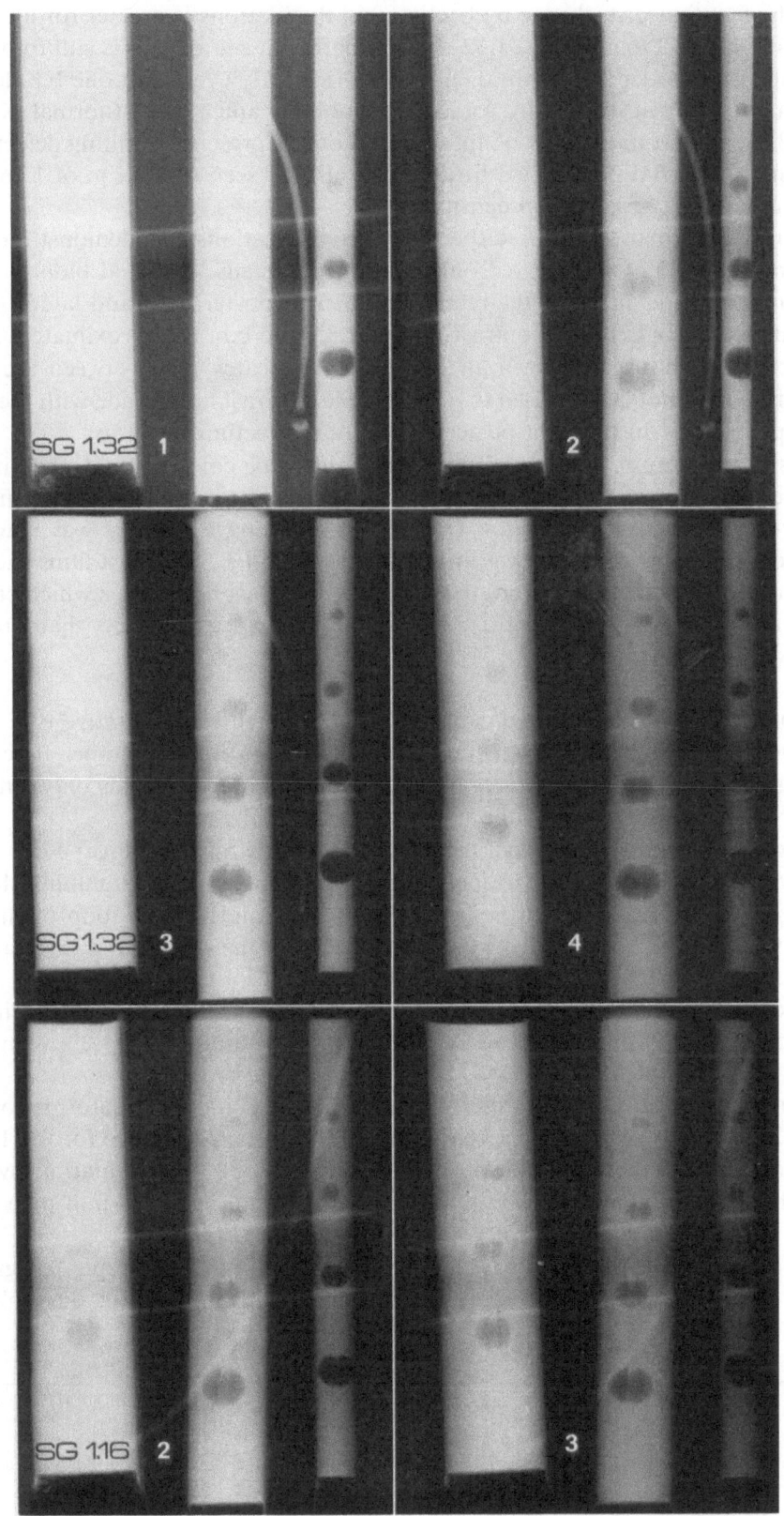

Fig. 14

In spite of the fact that disturbance by background fluctuations is greater for a contrast fluid with a s.g. of 1.16 and a b.b. 3 than for the 1.32–4 combination, a s.g. of 1.16 is still to be preferred since in the larger pipe the wooden beads are then seen more clearly even with one b.b. less. In practice, the combination of a contrast fluid with a s.g. of 1.32 or higher and a b.b. 1 (normal exposure) is generally used. Fig. 13 shows that in this way no information on the presence of filling defects is obtained in the large pipe and in the thin pipe only a little. It can also be seen that a s.g. of 1.16 obviously gives us more information for the same film density.

The practical confirmation of these theoretical considerations was demonstrated nicely with films of the rectum of a patient who visited our department because of rectal blood loss. Fig. 15A shows that the filling exposures made of the rectum in anterior-posterior, ¾ and lateral projection revealed no abnormalities. The s.g. of the contrast fluid is 1.32; the b.b. is approximately 2.

The difference in contrast between air and tissue is greater than between the contrast fluid and tissue so that we need not be surprised that the double-contrast films made with the same b.b. revealed a large polypoid tumor in the right posterior wall of the rectum (fig. 15D).

New films of the rectum were again made using the same contrast fluid, this time however with a b.b. of approximately 4 and 5. On these films, the polypoid tumor can be seen (fig. 15B).

Finally after thorough evacuation, a third series of filling exposures was made. The s.g. of the contrast fluid was 1.16 and the b.b. was approximately 2 and 3. These last films show the filling defect in the rectum very clearly. In addition, the contours of the sigmoid loops which cross each other can be followed more easily with the contrast medium of lower specific gravity than on the first two series of exposures (fig. 15c).

The two pipes with the contrast fluid can only be considered representative of a colon which is not too wide and for filling of the duodenum and the jejunum in the manner described in this study (duodenal intubation). The ileum however is less wide and mucosal folds only 2 mm thick must also be visible over their entire length without overexposure of the margins.

Furthermore small ulcers, diverticula and fistulous tracts may not escape our attention. The test procedure was therefore expanded to include a 14 mm plastic pipe containing the 4 wooden beads described previously. This pipe can be considered representative of a loop of the ileum. Finally, a thin plastic tube with a 2 mm lumen was introduced into the phantom such that it crossed several barium columns.

The 3 pipes and the tube were successively filled with contrast fluids with specific gravities of 1.16 and 1.32. For s.g. 1.16, films were made with b.b. 2 and 3 and for s.g. 1.32, with b.b. 1, 2, 3, and 4 (fig. 14).

It is striking that for this series of experiments the greatest amount of information is again obtained with s.g. 1.32 and b.b. 4 or with s.g. 1.16 and b.b. 3. Here the preference for the 1.16–3 combination is greater than in the other experiments because for the 1.32–4 combination overexposure almost occurs for the 2 mm tube and the density of the largest bead in the 14 mm pipe is so high that the central hole is no longer clearly visible.

With a contrast fluid with a s.g. of 1.32, the information in the 'ileum pipe' is greater with a b.b. 3 than with a b.b. 4, the tube is also more clearly visible with b.b. 3. For the 'colon pipe' the lower

Fig. 15
Visibility of polypoid mass in rectum under various exposure conditions.
A: s.g. contrast fluid 1.32   B.b. 2
B: s.g. contrast fluid 1.32   B.b. 4—5
C: s.g. contrast fluid 1.16   B.b. 2—3
D: double contrast exposures B.b. 2

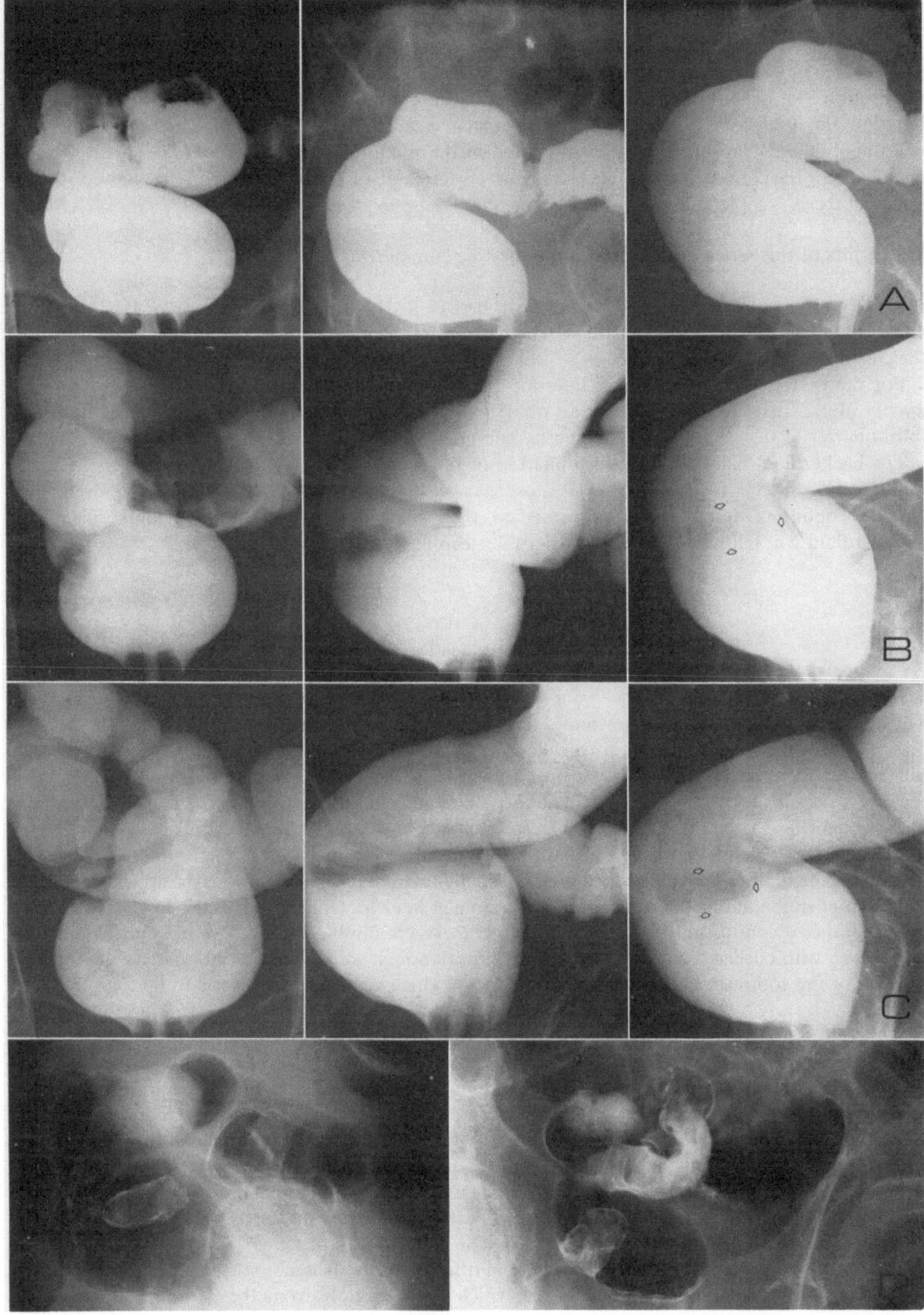

specific gravity was usually to be preferred; it is therefore sensible to be guided by this factor so that for less wide loops, the density can be decreased from 3 to 2 without loss of information, which means a reduction in dosage for the patient. Although the tube is most clearly visible with the 1.32–2 combination, the opacification caused by the two smaller beads in the 'jejunum pipe' is too vague.

Probably the best results for the examination of the small intestine will be obtained with a b.b. 2 and a s.g. for the contrast fluid somewhere between 1.16 and 1.32. Practical experience has confirmed this hypothesis completely.

The results of this series of experiments can best be summarized as follows:

For a colon examination, a contrast fluid can best be used with a specific gravity of 1.15 for a thin and at the most 1.2 for an obese patient. The background blackening must lie in the upper fourth of the steep part of the density curve.

For the examination of the small intestine, a contrast medium can best be used with a specific gravity of 1.2 for a thin and 1.25 for an obese patient. The background blackening must lie in the third quarter of the steep part of the density curve.

The background blackening for examination of the digestive tract may therefore never lie in the lower half of the density curve.

If the conditions described here are satisfied, then blackening of the intestinal loops filled with contrast fluid will fall in the lower fourth of the steep part of the density curve.

7. Comparative studies with different brands

For the past 40 years, comparative studies have formed the basis for diverse radiologists for chosing one of the various brands of contrast media (175, 203). These studies were often the direct result of the fact that the preparations used were unsatisfactory. There is no purpose in repeating the names of the diverse brands used in these tests; since then many have disappeared from the market and others have probably appeared in a new form. The contrast media chosen for these tests also depended upon the brands available at that time; in addition the results obtained were directly influenced by the nature and methods of the studies themselves. Usually the rate of sedimentation, the adhesion and the stability under conditions of changing pH were studied in vitro. Only a few studies in vivo have been reported; then 2 contrast media were compared by means of double examination of adults with sprue or children with coeliac disease (7, 8, 57). Significant enough to be worth mentioning is the marked stability of the contrast medium Raybar (Demancy), which according to reports in literature cannot be matched by any other brand. Mixobar (Astra) is apparently also quite stable (165). Many radiologists therefore use Raybar for the second examination of patients with the malabsorption syndrome when flocculation has occurred during the first examination with the contrast medium normally used. The manufacturer of Raybar states that the adhesive characteristics of this exceedingly stable contrast medium are obviously not as good as those of Micropaque, which they also produce and which is recommended for routine examinations. We have also found that there is little reason to be satisfied with the adhesive characteristics of Mixobar; we have not had enough experience with Raybar. Others have compared in vitro pure barium sulfate with one or more preparations which were highly satisfactory in vivo. As a result, we have gained better understanding of the importance of adding substances to enhance stability. In this respect, the experiments of BRAECKMAN (22), ZIMMER (224) and BROWN (24) are the most valuable to be found in literature. It is not surprising that many have considered the possibility of contrast media which differ entirely from the barium sulfate. These will be discussed in the following chapter. Comparative studies however were only carried out for barium and Gastrografine; for these tests, barium was to be preferred in almost all respects.

8. Contrast media other than barium sulfate

BARIUM CARBONATE

In 1959 the gastric examination of a number of patients was carried out using barium carbonate. In 8 patients there were severe symptoms of poisoning, including cyanosis, irregular heart activity, intestinal complaints and paresis. In the 6 patients who died as a result, autopsy revealed a hemorrhagic infiltration of the meninges and cerebral edema. Before the barium carbonate had been administered to patients, extensive animal experiments had been carried out and no ill-effects had been found (128).

DISADVANTAGES OF BARIUM SUSPENSIONS

In addition to the great difficulties still encountered in producing a sufficiently stable barium suspension which is at the same time protected against fluid withdrawal, several other disadvantages of this contrast medium are mentioned in literature.

1. owing to the higher viscosity of a barium suspension in the ileum, it cannot deeply penetrate narrow fistulous tracts in this area.
2. as a result of leakage from perforations or fistulas, the formation of barium granulomas can occur.
3. as a result of aspiration, a necrotizing bronchopneumonia can develop.

Some radiologists have therefore tried to find a contrast medium which does not have these disadvantages. They considered organic iodine compounds since the thin liquid aqueous iodine solutions are just as unsatisfactory; this will be discussed in more detail in this chapter.

SUSPENSIONS OF AN ORGANIC IODINE COMPOUND

JONES et al. (99) studied tetraiodophtalimidoethanol; they were able to produce a very homogeneous suspension with a particle size of 1–2 microns. This fluid contains 73 per cent iodine, barely precipitates and adheres more readily to the mucosa then barium suspensions. By adding gelatin, the characteristics of the suspension were further improved. From animal experiments it appeared that the toxicity of this contrast medium is as low as that of barium sulfate; for the latter it has been shown that particles varying from 0.04 to 0.1 microns in size can be absorbed by the intestinal mucous membrane. These particles, which do not end up in the blood stream but in the lymphatic channels, form less than one ten-thousandth of the normal barium suspension (4). The organic iodine compounds were tested in several experiments with dogs; it appeared that much smaller mucosal lesions could be localized with this contrast medium than with barium.

In 18 patients and a number of students, a total of 56 follow-through studies and 4 colon examinations were carried out. The resulting roentgenograms were very clear. One objection was that fluid absorption in the distal ileum and the colon caused even greater dehydration of the contrast fluid than barium. Unfortunately the preparation of this contrast medium was so time-consuming and expensive that the experiments had to be terminated.

AQUEOUS IODINE SOLUTIONS

In 1958, the first publications appeared on the use of Urokon, Hypaque and Renographin as contrast media for examination of the digestive tract. Shortly thereafter, similar articles were also published in England and Germany. A true avalanche of reports from enthusiastic users broke loose after the introduction of Gastrografine about 1960. After Gastrografine, which consists of 76 per cent Urografine mixed with a wetting agent, a sweetener and a flavoring, several other brands were introduced but they have never been generally accepted. Most radiologists believed that Gastrografine was ideal for use when barium fails due to flocculation or when barium is contra-indicated. The following examples of the latter are mentioned:

1. atresia or fistulas in the tracheo-esophageal area (danger of aspiration).
2. special cases of pre- and post-operative diagnosis of the digestive tract, such as bleeding ulcers, suture leakage or perforations.
3. partial obstructions which cannot be passed by barium or where dehydration and thickening of the barium suspension might occur.

There were however also publications reporting the use of Gastrografine for all patients, for the colon examination as well as the examinations of the stomach and the small intestine. SHEHADI even reports a series of 1500 patients (191). ROBINSON and LEVENE (181) prefer Renografin over barium for the gastro-intestinal examination. In 1959, LESSMAN and LILIENFELD (121) had already studied and compared the experiences of various radiologists. It appeared that the amount of Gastrografine used per examination varied widely. Some used only 25–50 ml of a 76 per cent concentration and others used 10 times as much. There was general satisfaction with the reproduction of the gastric mucosal relief and the greater ease with which a pyloric stenosis could be diagnosed or a fistulous tract filled. However they all discovered that dilution of the contrast medium in the small intestine was so great that morphological evaluation of this area was absolutely impossible. In addition, no-one succeeded in making acceptable double-contrast exposures; and some authors report that more than 50 ml can cause abdominal cramps, vomiting and diarrhea. Reasonably satisfactory colon films can be made because absorption of fluid causes an increasing contrast in this area (191). In this way it was often possible to obtain good filling of the colon on the proximal side of a stenosis which could not be passed by the barium from the distal side. It remained impossible to localize tumors in the small intestine, although the diagnosis 'obstruction' could often be made on the basis of the presence of wide loops.

Some radiologists believe that when the Gastrografine has not yet reached the colon 4 hours after oral administration, a post-operative ileus is due to an obstruction and not a paralysis (210).

RUBIN et al. (183) were not able to confirm this opinion. BERGER of Philadelphia agrees with RUBIN and at a conference he showed slides of 4 patients. In these cases the Gastrografine was visible in the colon within 15 minutes although a definite obstruction did exist in the small intestine which apparently could easily be passed by the thin liquid Gastrografine. In approximately 2 per cent of the patients, some of the iodine contrast medium is excreted into the urine (86). This is believed by some to indicate an obstruction, perforation or other pathological condition in the digestive tract (148). Although surgical confirmation has often supported this line of thought and TOSCH has shown with radioactive Gastrografine that this can indeed occur (208), disappointments (220) and false positive results have also been reported in this respect (182). In 1959, LESSMAN and LILIENFELD already pointed out the strong hyperosmotic characteristics of Gastrografine and the dangers this can cause for intestinal obstructions (121). Since the osmotic value of 50 ml 70 per cent Urokon is equal to that of 15 g magnesium sulfate, a dose of 6 ml per kg body weight can cause such excessive fluid withdrawal that the circulating plasma volume can decrease 15–30 per cent. HARRIS et al. have described lethal complications in children due to the hypovolemia. They also showed that the osmotic force of Gastrografine in isolated intestinal loops can be so great that blood circulation in the intestinal wall can be seriously disturbed (81). In addition the vomiting and diarrhea caused by Gastrografine can further disturb an already critical electrolyte balance (156). It has therefore become clear that for cases of suspected obstruction in the small intestine it is far from certain that Gastrografine is the most suitable contrast medium. If considered desirable, then it must in any event be handled with extreme caution and used only when the clinical condition of the patient permits it. Furthermore when Gastrografine is used, it must be realized that this contrast medium does not adhere easily and therefore reliable morphological information can only be obtained when filling is complete. In addition Gastrografine is such a thin liquid that fistulous tracts or perforations may not be discovered because the contrast medium passes so rapidly that there is not enough time for penetration.

SHEHADI wrote in 1960 that the introduction of the aqueous iodine contrast medium could be considered a milestone in the diagnosis of the digestive tract (192). Fortunately since then application of Gastrografine has lost some of the ground it had taken by storm; however a new landmark in the diagnosis of the digestive tract will be reached when use of this medium is only a rare exception.

GASTROGRAFINE-BARIUM MIXTURES

A number of radiologists did not simply stop using Gastrografine but have attempted to obtain better results by mixing it with barium (70, 202). They expected the mixture to have the better adhesive characteristics of a barium suspension on the one hand, and the transit acceleration and the ability to mix with gastric and intestinal juices without flocculation of Gastrografine on the other. The combination of these two entirely different contrast fluids was tested in every possible ratio, especially in Japan where it is still used extensively for gastric and duodenal examinations. During these tests it appeared that the tendency of barium to flocculate does not decrease; it even increases as the amount of barium in the mixture decreases. The transit acceleration of the Gastrografine-barium mixture does not depend particularly on the ratio but is almost directly dependent upon the absolute quantity of Gastrografine.

Both SHEHADI (191) and STECKEN et al. (202) report the strange phenomenon of separation of barium and Gastrografine already occurring in the jejunum. The Gastrografine produces less contrast as a result of the absorption of fluid and it travels rapidly to the cecum while the barium remains in the jejunum. Furthermore STECKEN et al. observed that not only stenosis and hypotonia but also meteorism clearly delay the rate of transit. Various radiologists believe that 150 ml barium suspension and approximately 30 ml Gastrografine is still the most satisfactory ratio. This is probably because there is so little Gastrografine in this mixture that it barely affects the barium suspension; furthermore it is not impossible that the 30 ml Gastrografine does not visibly separate from the barium in the duodenum and the jejunum and absorbs sufficient fluid to cause transit acceleration. Due to the faster transit a larger portion of the intestine can be photographed with the still usable barium suspension then would otherwise be the case.

VI
METHODS OF EXAMINATION

In the previous chapter we have seen that even today only barium sulfate qualifies as contrast medium for the examination of the small intestine. As a result of the numerous additives however it is still not easy to make the proper choice.

In this chapter we shall see that for the methods of examination the situation is not much better; the differences between these methods are presumably even greater than between the contrast media. The combination of these choices finally determines the result we shall obtain and this can indeed vary from very good to very bad.

1. 'Physiological' examination of the small intestine

In Chapter II it was noted that addition of nutrients to the contrast medium was abandoned during the second world war. The problems involved in the functional examination were found to be considerably greater than those for the morphological examination. Furthermore it was recognized that a functional examination must also be evaluated morphologically. It is therefore necessary that the morphological examination of the small intestine first attain a much higher degree of perfection. In the sixties, only MATTSSON et al. (45, 140) advocated a return to this method. As mentioned previously (p. 29), the pictures of the ileum on their published photographs were very poor. The nutritional composition of the 300 ml contrast meal is approximately the same as Borgström's and is as follows:

153 g $BaSO_4$
$12\frac{1}{2}$ g protein
15 g fat
$12\frac{1}{2}$ g lactose
25 g dextrose
200 ml water.

In one of their articles they report that their examination technique gave very constant transit times, in contrast to the highly variable data from literature. The authors hereby show that they have no insight into the reasons for these variations.

It is customary for many radiologists to give their patients sooner or later something to eat or drink whenever a standstill of the contrast column has occurred in the ileum; this has of course nothing to do with a physiological examination. This additional food is usually given to renew stimulation of the peristalsis, sometimes however only to remove the patient's feeling of hunger.

Some radiologists have set rules; PIRK and VULTERINOVÁ (166) for instance give a small meal after 3 hours if the stomach is empty and the cecum has not yet been reached. Patients with gastric resections even receive this food after 2 hours. When this is done, we must realize that a large, liquid meal will induce more active peristalsis and faster transit than a small, more viscous meal. In the first case, therefore, the chance will be greater that additional food will disturb the contrast pictures in the ileum, in so far as this has not already occurred as a result of the long transit time.

2. Single administration of the contrast medium

NORMAL AMOUNT

For examination of the small intestine, most radiologists including GOLDEN have the patient drink approximately 250 ml of the contrast fluid. Usually this is preceded by a gastric examination whereby the mucosa is studied using approximately 50 ml contrast fluid. The number of exposures susbsequently made of the small intestine is highly dependent upon the rate of transit but possibly even more upon the attitude of the radiologist. Many are in the habit of making films at equal time intervals even when the rate of transit continues to decrease. This of course is not correct, in this case the patient receives an unnecessarily high radiation dosage and in addition, it means a waste of film material.

There is no waste of film material for those who believe that an examination of the many meters of small intestine can be carried out with only 3 (221) or even 2 (150) exposures. It is not necessary to demonstrate that this method is very dangerous and therefore should be rejected, even when each of these exposures clearly shows practically the entire small intestine.

SMALL AMOUNTS

Some radiologists use small quantities of contrast fluid, such as LAWS et al. who administer only 100 ml undiluted Micropaque even for sprue patients (114). This is probably done to avoid the annoying effect of superposition, but this exaggerated fear must be paid for with flocculation and segmentation. MORTON, who only used 70 g Micropaque powder mixed with 200 ml of an ice-cold physiological salt solution (150), also obtained poor results. He made only 2 exposures, but probably the information would not be increased by an increase in this number.

LARGE AMOUNTS

For many years, an increasing number of radiologists have switched over to the use of large quantities of the contrast medium for examination of the small intestine.

Although there was no response, WELTZ in 1937 had already pointed out that the quality of the contrast films of the small intestine is highly dependent upon the degree of filling (214). He also reported that this requires rapid gastric emptying and that stretching of the small intestine is the main stimulus for the induction of good peristaltic waves. Furthermore he believed that a large amount of contrast medium offers the best buffer action against the detrimnetal effects of secretion and absorption in the intestinal canal. He had noted that the contrast intensity in the ileum is greater than in the jejunum but that this phenomenon is less pronounced for a rapid transit because there is apparently not enough time for fluid absorption.

In view of the time in which he worked, his insights can be regarded as brilliant. If he had had a better 'sales technique', the development of the radiological examination of the small intestine would certainly have advanced much further.

According to the articles published, MARSHAK had similar views but did not reason them as well as WELTZ. In any event, MARSHAK's great contribution was that these improvements in the examination technique were widely published in his numerous articles since 1954 (132–138). He routinely used 480 ml contrast fluid and when the small intestine was dilated, sometimes 600 ml or more (137).

In 1963, CALDWELL and FLOCH examined 32 patients twice and thereby showed that the transit time is significantly shorter when the amount of contrast medium is chosen according to MARSHAK (480 ml) rather than GOLDEN (240 ml). For the former, the average transit time was 2.25 hours and for the latter, 3.25 hours (31).

Many authors believe that it is desirably to make compression exposures of the ileum, whereby the loops which cover one another are forced aside (132, 201).

Numerous radiologists also find that diagnosis is considerably improved when several exposures are made, one immediately after the other; the same intestinal loops are then seen more often in approximately the same stage of filling (217, 221). CALDWELL et al. (32) pointed out that a delayed gastric emptying can still cause flocculation and segmentation even when 500 ml stable barium is administered.

It is striking that none of the radiologists who use large quantities of the contrast medium feel the need of either ice water or accelerators.

3. Fractional administration of the contrast medium

METHOD OF PANSDORF

In 1927 PANSDORF (159) had already introduced this method based on the entirely reasonable assumption that the best technique for administering the contrast medium must be extreme fractionation. He gave his patients one tablespoon to drink every 5 minutes and thought that only in this way could distribution of the contrast medium throughout the small intestinal loops be guaranteed; furthermore the annoying effect of superposition would be very slight, at the most. He reasoned that each roentgenogram would then show as many loops as possible.

PANSDORF was probably not sufficiently aware of the numerous factors which can completely disturb this theoretically uniform supply. Ideal fractionation only exists when administration of the contrast medium is matched by gastric emptying through the pyloric canal (fig. 16 and p. 57). In addition the stability of the contrast medium is too low to be able to withstand such an unfavourable ratio with respect to the intestinal fluids. It is however possible that at the time of PANSDORF, this technique of fractional administration of the contrast medium was not as unfavourable as now. After all, the contrast medium then used was highly unstable even without the addition of food and disintegration occurred anyway in the proximal part of the intestine. Possibly a distribution of flocculation or segmentation was still to be preferred over large segment clumps. Should there ever be completely stable contrast media in the future, then it is conceivable that the principle of fractional administration will regain a place of honor.

MODIFICATION OF WELTZ

In 1937, WELTZ (214) introduced important changes in the method of Pansdorf by first giving a single dose of 200 ml contrast medium for the gastric examination. For the subsequent follow-through study, the patient drank approximately 30 ml every 5 minutes. As mentioned previously (p. 45), WELTZ

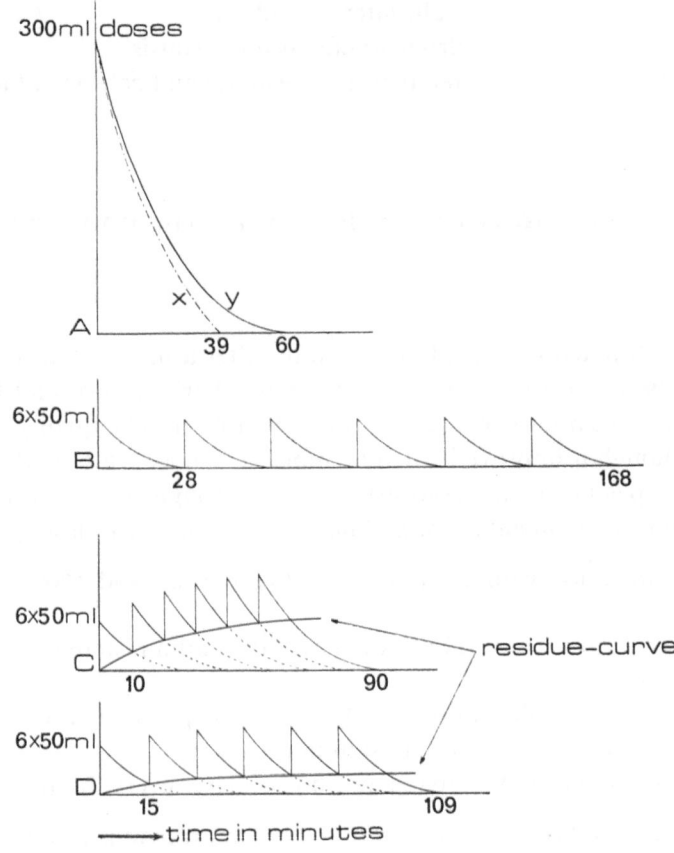

Fig. 16
A: Gastric emptying curve
   y: sitting or standing position————
   x: right lateral position–.–.–
B: Ideal fractionation: rate of supply equals rate of emptying
C, D: Fractionation: rate of supply is greater than rate of emptying so
that an increasing residual is found in the stomach.

believed in a large dosage of contrast medium. Although his method appears to resemble fractionation, this is in fact not true. The stomach is continuously filled to a large extent and fractionation is probably only meant to keep the patient from feeling that his stomach is much too full.

MODIFICATION OF NAUMANN

NAUMANN (154) administered two doses of 200 ml a half hour apart. Again this method cannot be regarded as true fractionation; it is used to administer a slightly larger amount of contrast medium without discomfort to the patient.

FRACTIONATION BY THE PYLORIC MUSCLE

It is probably useful to realize that every quantity of contrast medium administered orally is passed on to the small intestine in fractions by the pylorus. The dosage of these fractions differs for every patient and is partly dependent upon:

pylorus function   right lateral position
peptic ulcer or tumor   drugs to enhance peristalsis
gastric acid concentration   temperature, osmotic and caloric value of the contrast fluid.

4. Administration of cold fluids with the contrast medium

METHOD OF WEINTRAUB AND WILLIAMS

In 1941 WEINTRAUB (213) noted that drinking ice water after a meal enhanced peristalsis and caused diarrhea. Using this observation he gave ice water after a barium meal and found that in about 50 per cent of the cases, the cecum was reached within a half hour. The quality of the pictures however was not very good although it improved when he replaced the ice water with cold physiological salt. It was remarkable that passage of the contrast medium through the small intestine proceeded even more rapidly. After some experimentation, he finally settled on the following technique:

1. gastro-duodenal examination with a mixture of 120 g barium and 120 g isotonic salt solution at room temperature.
2. after this examination, 240 g ice-cold physiological salt is administered and after 5 minutes, a new roentgenogram is made.
3. immediately after this x-ray film, another 240 g ice-cold physiological salt is administered and again a new roentgenogram is made after 10 minutes.
4. 15 minutes later, still another film is made and fi necessary, every 30 minutes afterward.

As a result of the large amount of fluid given in total (700 ml) transit is rapid and the barium does not thicken in the ileum. He even reports that when the transit time is short, the quality of the films is good and it is poor when the transit time is longer. It is understandable that this method of examination is not very pleasant for the patients.

SIMPLIFIED VARIATIONS

GOLDEN found the method of Weintraub too arduous and believed in addition that the great haste involved was not opportune since precise following and evaluation of the transit films already cost so much time. Many other authors also found this method of examination too laborious but they did want to profit from the passage acceleration caused bij a cold liquid. The simplifications introduced are so similar that they will not be discussed as separate modifications.

ETTINGER (47) gave a glass of ice water after first examining the stomach with a mixture of 120 g barium and 120 ml water. HUDAK (92) administered a glass of ice-cold physiological salt solution 10 minutes after a small barium meal and 10 minutes later, 1 mg prostigmin.

BENDICK (14) gave 200 ml ice-cold soda water after the contrast meal. He had noted that the gas formation which is then caused induces peristalsis. We have already seen (p. 13) that this gas travels to the cecum rapidly and completely independently and therefore certainly does not accelerate passage of the contrast medium. Apparently BROWN's experiences were similar (23). In spite of the fact that he even gave 3 glasses of ice-cold soda water, in only 60 per cent of his patients had the cecum been reached within 2 hours. He tried to prevent the pronounced flocculation and segmentation of the contrast fluid which then occur by using Raybar, the most stable contrast medium known. MORTON (150) gave the patient a mixture of 200 ml ice-cold salt solution and only 70 g Micropaque powder. Like those of HUDAK, his photographs show only flocculation and segmentation of the contrast fluid and therefore demonstrate quite clearly how unsuitable this technique is.

All the authors in this group report a transit time to the cecum of 1.5 to 2 hours, thus considerably longer than with the method of Weintraub. No-one apparently recognized the importance of the large quantities; they all used 200 ml instead of 700 ml like WEINTRAUB. In this connection it is very interesting to note the technique of BROWN who did give approximately 600 ml fluid. The passage acceleration which this large dosage should have produced was completely neutralized by the retardation caused by the development of gas.

5. Administration of the contrast medium through a tube directly into the small intestine (enteroclysis)

Publications between 1920 and 1925 by EINHORN, who introduced the contrast fluid into the duodenum through a tube and obtained outstanding films, gave PESQUERA the idea in 1929 of using this method for filling the entire small intestine (164). He administered a mixture of barium and water, also containing a small amount of gum acacia. Although no quantities are reported, the article indicates that he let the infusion run slowly as long as necessary to reach the cecum, usually no longer than half an hour. He reports that he was able to diagnose a lymphosarcoma in the distal ileum in this manner; this can certainly be regarded as a success in radiological diagnosis at that time.

Ten years later, GERSHON-COHEN and SHAY (64) did some experiments on the function of the pylorus and noted that the closing mechanism was very good. After the duodenum had been filled using a tube, the entire contents quickly disappeared into the jejunum; reflux into the stomach occurred only when the pressure of the infusion was too high. They used this method to administer 800–1200 ml contrast fluid and they were surprised by the rapid rate of transit through the small intestine. The cecum was reached in 8–15 minutes. This interval would probably have been even shorter if the pressure of the infusion had been higher; their level difference was only 25 cm.

In 1943, a publication by SCHATZKI (185) appeared reporting on 75 patients examined in this manner. He intubated a supple Rehfuss tube with an olive-shaped metal end into the duodenum and let 500–1000 ml barium suspension with a lower specific gravity than he normally used for a gastric examination run through this tube. In half of his patients the cecum was reached in 15 min. For 4 patients, reflux into the stomach occurred; in these cases the average transit time was more than 40 minutes, thus considerably longer. The rather low percentage of reflux and the relatively long transit time for such an examination with large amounts of contrast fluid probably indicate that his infusion was given under low pressure.

Once reflux into the stomach had occurred, SCHATZKI tried to end it by sliding the tube further into the duodenum, decreasing the pressure of the infusion or acidifying the barium mixture. He was not successful with any of these methods, so that he concluded that these factors do not influence the development of reflux. The correctness of this conclusion is however very doubtful since it is obvious that once reflux has occurred, the pylorus will continue to open to allow the gastric contents to pass on to the duodenum. While the infusion is flowing, the pressure in the duodenum will probably be higher than in the stomach and opening of the pylorus will therefore have a reverse effect.

SCHATZKI's great contribution is that he pointed out the importance of administering large quantities of the contrast medium in the right lateral position. He had found that interruption of the contrast column lengthens the transit time considerably, thus allowing more time for dehydration in the ileum.

In 1951 LURA (125) reported on a series of 300 patients; he examined the small intestine of these patients using the infusion technique and found an average transit time of 15 minutes. It had been difficult to pass the tube through the pylorus in 5–10 per cent of the cases.

In 1960 SCOTT HARDEN et al. (110, 187) and PYGOTT et al. (173) described an improvement in the technique for duodenal intubation. They passed 2 catheters one inside the other into the pars media of the stomach; which can be felt as well as seen by fluoroscopy since the outer end of both catheters is marked by a metal ring. The outer more rigid catheter has an outer diameter of 5.8 mm and the inner more pliable catheter has a lumen 1.5 mm in diameter. The inner catheter is then slid through the outer into the pyloric canal. It appeared that curling of the catheter could often be prevented by placing the patient in the right lateral position.

In spite of this simplification of the technique, they were still not able to get the catheter into the duodenum in 7 per cent of the patients, which must be considered a high percentage. We have found that beginning this procedure with the more rigid catheter was probably the reason for their failure.

Both catheters remain in place, only the end of the inner catheter with the narrow lumen lies in the duodenum. PYGOTT et al. then used a syringe to administer 50 ml contrast fluid into the duodenum as often as necessary. It is possible that as a result continuity of the contrast column is occasionally interrupted and probably the outflow through this narrow lumen is too low to cause sufficient stretching of the duodenal wall to induce good peristalsis.

SCOTT HARDEN administered only 80 ml of a thin Microtrast solution, directly followed by a MgSO$_4$ solution. It is clear that this method will certainly not lead to good results since both the hyperosmotic MgSO$_4$ solution and the low dosage of contrast medium induce marked flocculation.

In 1965, PATTERSON et al. (160) reported that they had injected 40 ml Raybar in 15 sprue patients through a duodenal tube. Fifteen minutes later they administered 500 ml ice water as well as a MgSO$_4$ solution. Obviously they obtained flocculation in this manner even with this exceedingly stable contrast medium. Here we are confronted not only with an actual abuse of a good examination technique but also with an entirely misplaced conclusion drawn from their experiments: 'for sprue, an examination technique of duodenal intubation offers no advantages over oral administration of the contrast medium'. It is noteworthy that orally they did not give 40 ml Raybar with ice water and MgSO$_4$, as would be expected, but 120 g undiluted Micropaque solution!

The only techniques which might be regarded as a variation of the preceeding are those of GREEN-SPON (78) and FRIEDMAN and RIGLER (60). In 1960 they reported that they introduced a triple-lumen Miller-Abbott tube (fig. 17) into the small intestine just beyond the area they wished to examine.

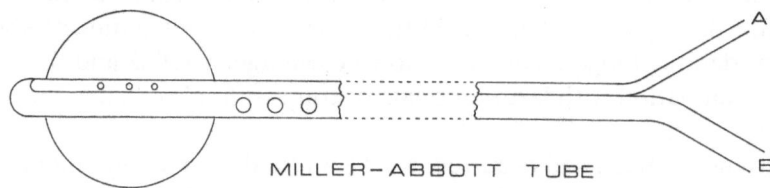

MILLER-ABBOTT TUBE

Fig. 17
A: air inflow. B: contrast fluid

It can take several days for the end of the tube to reach the desired location. The balloon is filled with 50 to 60 ml air through tube A so that passage beyond this location is not possible. Contrast fluid is then administered through tube B. In this way, according to the authors, one-fourth of the small intestine can be examined without the annoying effect of superposition. Because the intestine is suddenly occluded, the patients cannot easily tolerate more than 600 ml contrast medium. Abdominal cramps can also be caused when the contrast fluid is injected too quickly or its temperature is too low. It is clear that this method of examination is not suitable for routine use and is probably also seldom necessary.

6. Retrograde administration of the contrast fluid

In the twenties and thirties, some authors believed (correctly) that it is better to examine the distal ileum using the colon enema technique rather than the small intestine transit examination.

Although the situation had changed somewhat in 1964, FIGIEL and FIGIEL (49) pointed out that retrograde filling of the ileum could still mean a welcome supplement to the transit examination for the diagnosis of strictures, adhesions, ulcerations, fistulas and diverticula. They demonstrated this with the x-rays of a number of patients examined in this manner. They found abnormalities which were confirmed surgically while the normal transit examination had revealed nothing.

MILLER (144, 146) found that especially in the ileum the intestinal appearance is determined by peristalsis and tone to such a large extent that constricting lesions in an early stage and smaller mucosal lesions are definitely missed during a transit examination. The function of the pylorus causes intermittant, irregular and incomplete fillings so that the elasticity of the intestine cannot be determined. Furthermore flocculation and segmentation often completely distort the evaluation.

MILLER finds enteroclysis a good method of examination but the duodenal intubation beforehand too troublesome. He propagates retrograde filling of the entire small intestine. Although it is possible to reach the stomach in 9 out of 10 patients, he advises terminating the filling of the small intestine as the duodenum is approached. It is obvious that this filling must occur under fluoroscopic control and that one must be careful that the contrast fluid does not enter the lungs by way of the stomach and esophagus. Passing the valve of Bauhin causes difficulties in 4 per cent of the patients, which can be prevented by oral administration of 1 mg atropine before the examination; this also decreases the secretion of intestinal juices.

The amount of contrast medium needed to fill the colon and small intestine is sometimes less than 2 liters, sometimes considerably more. More than 4.5 liters are never given, even if the duodenum has not yet been reached.

MILLER later changed this method slightly by replacing the barium suspension with a physiological salt solution as soon as the ileum begins to fill. When the infusion of the contrast medium is terminated, the colon is quickly emptied by first placing the plastic infusion bag below the level of the table and then sending the patient to the toilet for about 30 seconds. Films of the small intestine are subsequently made; because of the rapid emptying, the radiologist does not have much time. If desired of course, films of the colon can be made at the beginning of the infusion period.

For this examination, MILLER advises a stable barium suspension with a specific gravity which is not too high.

An enormous advantage of this method is that stenotic processes in the small intestine can be approached very quickly from the distal direction. Proximal approach in these cases costs more time and moreover an annoying dilution of the contrast medium can occur in the dilated loops.

7. Combined methods of examination

Without a doubt, many radiologists use methods which are not described here or which are made up of elements or variations of specific methods of examination.

An example of such a combination is the approach of BUGYI (27), who first examines the gall bladder and stomach according to the method of GIANTURCO (68), then the small intestine using a variation of the method of WEINTRAUB and finally takes pictures of the orally-filled colon.

The following procedures occur in the given order:

1. On the morning of the examination, gall bladder photographs are taken first. On the afternoon of the previous day the patient swallowed the necessary tablets.
2. After the gall bladder photographs are taken, the colon is cleansed by means of an enema.
3. The next step is the gastric examination. No details are given.
4. After the gastric examination, the patient receives 100–200 g paraffin oil, which is a laxative and also induces contraction of the gall bladder.
5. A half hour later, photographs of the contracted gall bladder are taken.
6. Patient is given a glass of ice-cold salt solution.
7. Films of the small intestine are now made every 10 minutes.
8. 4–6 hours after the beginning of the examination, films are made of the orally-filled colon.

Unfortunately the article contains no photographs of his results. BUGYI suffices with the statement that he is highly satisfied with this method and that a colon enema examination only occurs upon strict indications.

8. Laxation before the examination and the use of the right lateral position

Many radiologists are accustomed to enhancing gastric emptying by having the patient lie on his right side.

PRÉVÔT, even in 1940, appears to have used this method (171); in the sixties it is reported by FRIEDEN-BERG et al. (58), CALDWELL et al. (32) and NICE (157), as well as others. NICE measured the transit time in 106 students. Unfortunately since this small number was used to study the influence of no less than 12 different factors, few conclusions can be drawn from this experiment. He did note however, also during a later experiment with 104 students, that in all groups the transit time was lengthened when the cecum was filled with feces. Drinking of a physiological salt solution and water after administration of the contrast medium decreased the quality of the mucosal patterns.

9. Use of drugs to accelerate transit

The radiologists' growing lack of time and the high demands on the patience and endurance of the patient are the reasons why shortening the length of the examination has been an objective for so many years. We have already seen that this can be accomplished by:

1. drinking very large quantities of contrast fluid.
2. administering the contrast fluid directly into the duodenum by infusion.
3. supplementary administration of cold fluids.
4. mixture of the contrast fluid with Gastrografine. The patient finds methods 1 and 2 more or less unpleasant; method 4 has an unfavourable effect on the quality of the image and method 3 combines both of these unpleasant characteristics.

In the past few years, several drugs which are in no way unpleasant for the patient have been used to increase the rate of transit. The effect of these drugs differs greatly; we shall discuss each of them briefly.

PROSTIGMIN

A substance long known for its accelerating effect on transit but used only seldom is neostigmine methylsulfate or prostigmin. In Chapter IV (p. 12), we have seen that this substance inhibits acetylcholinesterase so that the acetylcholine is protected against hydrolysis and can be active longer. The effective dosage for adults is 0.75–1.0 mg and for children, 0.25–0.5 mg. It can be administered subcutaneously, intramuscularly or intravenously; with the latter, the effect is the strongest but lasts only a few minutes. The effect of prostigmin can be neutralized by atropine.

Contra-indications for the use of prostigmin are: recent myocardial infarction, volvulus, invagination and complete obstruction or perforation of the small intestine. Prostigmin has no effect when there is dysfunction of the nerve cells, as in sprue.

An older publication on the use of this substance in a follow-through examination is that of HUDAK (92) in 1951. As a result of a combination of factors however, the intestinal appearances on the photographs published are very poor. HUDAK used only a small amount of contrast fluid (not specifically reported) and afterwards he even gave a glass of ice-cold physiological salt solution, which had to result in complete flocculation and segmentation of the contrast medium.

In 1962 FRIEDENBERG et al. (58) also found that, in a series of almost 500 patients, 400 ml ice-cold salt solution had the same effect of transit acceleration as 400 ml water with 0.5 mg prostigmin but that the quality of the mucosal patterns was better with the latter.

MARGULIS has used prostigmin for examination of the stomach and small intestine of many thousands of patients to his complete satisfaction (129, 130). As a result of the more active peristalsis, the gastric emptying time is approximately half as long. Therefore he saw a decrease in the percentage of examination of children with flocculation and segmentation. MÜLLER (151) published his experiences with neoserine in 97 patients; however 10 per cent of the cases showed side-effects of a respiratory or cardio-vascular nature. Like MARGULIS he also saw segmentation still develop in the ileum. Both radiologists believed that the tone was too high, presumably still reverting to GOLDEN's 'disordered motor function' theory. Much more likely is the following explanation which is based on personal observations: after the short effect of the intravenously injected prostigmin, a period of hypotonia and passage retardation develops which inevitably results in flocculation and segmentation of the contrast medium.

SORBITOL

In 1957 PORCHER and CAROLI (168) described the passage acceleration caused by 30 g Sorbitol without the development of hypersecretion and segmentation. The latter however is contested by many authors although it must be noted that an overdosage of Sorbitol or mixing with other substances often appears to be the reason for their poor results (127, 176).

Sorbitol is a glucose product (hexahydric alcohol) which is absorbed slowly and causes only a slight increase in the blood sugar curve. It has caloric value and is hyperosmotic which can cause less clear mucosal patterns. In previous chapters we have seen that other factors can also play an important role here, such as quantity, method of administration and composition of the contrast medium.

It is likely that the lowest effective dosage must be the best because a higher dosage will cause a linear increase in fluid absorption but a gradual decrease in acceleration of transit. It is therefore probably correct to use 10–20 g as advised by the manufacturer and not to increase to 30 g as some do (199). MANECKE and SCHMIDT (127) found the same; they obtained poor results with 20–30 ml Karion F (variation of Sorbitol) and only 20 ml barium suspension. With 5–10 ml Karion F the mucosal patterns were good, but there was only a slight acceleration of transit. As a compromise they gave their patients 10 ml Karion F at the beginning of the examination. One hour later, the patient received another supplementary dose of 20 ml after films of the ileum had first been made. Furthermore Sorbitol is both cholecystokinetic and cholagogic; these 2 characteristics again have a favourable and an unfavourable aspect. The transit acceleration caused by these substances is favourable, the flocculation is unfavourable (p. 23).

For SACK (184), the transit acceleration caused by gall was still the reason for enhancing contraction of the gall bladder for follow-through examinations. He gave his patients Diabenol, a mixture of 10 g Sorbitol and 4 g powdered egg but not before the stomach was almost half empty since Diabenol does accelerate transit but of course also retards gastric emptying (p. 16). In 20 per cent of the patients, the substance was not successful, usually because of insufficient contraction or absence of the gall bladder. The evening before the examination SACK prescribed a liquid diet and a laxative to cleanse the colon. The mucosal patterns of ileum and colon on the films published are of good quality: it is quite clear that the barium suspension has retained the proper viscosity because of the rapid transit time (30 min!). Unfortunately SACK does not provide any further data; it seems likely that the quantities and characteristics of the contrast medium administered contributed more to his good results than Diabenol.

METOCLOPRAMIDE (PRIMPERAN)

Since about 1966, metoclopramide has been used increasingly for transit acceleration. Because of its effect on the brain stem, this substance is supposed to activate and regulate the tone and peristalsis of the small intestine and the stomach without influencing the secretion. This substance can be administered both orally and by injection; the effective dose is 10–20 mg for an adult (1 ampule of 2 ml = 10 mg). Intravenous injection produces of course the quickest effect; within 5 minutes enhancement of peristalsis can already be seen clearly as both the number and depth of the peristaltic waves increase. We have found that the effect lasts only 15-20 minutes; however most radiologists report a slightly longer effective period (91, 94).

Diverse authors report that with Primperan (trade name) transit is accelerated to such a degree that the cecum is usually reached in 1 to 2 hours (94). In these publications it is striking that the contrast medium dosage is usually not mentioned although this factor is at least equally important for the transit time (31) (p. 16, 46).

Some authors are justifiably of the opinion that accelerated gastric emptying is an important factor for the transit acceleration caused by metoclopramide. HOWARTH (91) reports that the gastric emptying time is halved by Primperan.

Many also believe that the improvement in the mucosal patterns of the ileum can be ascribed to a decrease in dehydration of the contrast medium as a result of the acceleration of transit. It is strange that the dilatation of duodenum and proximal jejunum frequently seen by accelerated gastric emptying is often believed to be a decrease in tone.

The more active peristalsis of the stomach is a time-saving factor for the gastric-duodenal examination and in addition can be useful for duodenal intubation and for cinematographical examination of fixed and immobile sections of the gastric wall.

If it seems necessary to use a transit accelerating drug, metoclopramide (Primperan) appears to be the best choice at present. This preparation is not hydrophilic and, as a result of the accelerated gastric emptying, causes stretching of the duodenum and thus transit acceleration.

LAXATIVES

Laxatives have also been used occasionally to accelerate transit (48). When the effect of these preparations results from volume increase in the intestine by attraction of fluid, they will have a highly detrimental effect on the quality of the roentgenograms.

VII
REVIEW AND CONCLUSION

If we now try to coordinate the diverse information presented in the preceding chapters, we find that it is not very easy. The number of factors which seem to fulfil a more or less important role in obtaining optimum results is considerably greater for the examination of the small intestine than any other radiological examination.

It may not be so surprising, and can only be considered a normal human reaction, that the radiologist is generally not very interested in that part of his profession where he often falls short. On the other hand, many data from the previous chapters come from radiologists who felt differently; due to their work, it is now possible to classify these facts and draw conclusions. It will be obvious that this requires not only the good results obtained with specific methods; the mediocre and sometimes even the poor results of other methods have been just as helpful.

During the study of the copious literature it became evident that various radiologists in the past had already perceived certain facets of the examination of the small intestine which have turned out to be quite correct. Their significance was at that time often not appreciated so that they found no response and were often forgotten for many years.

With the exception of several details, it therefore appeared impossible and even unnecessary to add a fundamentally different concept to this long list of ideas. The contribution of this study therefore is predominantly the evaluation and coordination of the highly divergent results and experiences of numerous radiologists in the past. Often these data have turned out to be directly or indirectly important for the development of the radiological examination of the small intestine. It is certainly surprising that on the basis of the literature survey alone, a number of guide lines could be established for an examination which is technically the best and which provides us with a maximum in anatomical information. Our surprise was however even greater when it appeared that practical application resulted in such a time-saving examination as well as superior information in comparison to modern conventional methods that the latter is no longer feasible even for routine use.

For the examination of the small intestine, it should be realized that this organ is several meters long and lies convoluted in a small space. Owing to tone and peristalsis, the mucosal patterns of each intestinal section vary greatly in different phases.

The objective of the radiological examination is to signalize restrictions in the mobility of the mucosa and anatomical abnormalities of the intestinal wall in an early stage. When the contact between the contrast medium and the mucosa is good, abnormalities can easily be observed. One condition is of course that each intestinal section be shown on at least 2 exposures without superposition. It is often difficult to locate the related intestinal segments on various photographs so that it is wise to make two exposures in succession. In the case of hypertonic, contracted loops, the highly folded mucosa lies even more loosely over the innermost layers of the intestinal wall so that deeper abnormalities in this wall can be concealed completely. In general in a hypotonic or dilated intestine, abnormalities located outside the mucosa are seen more easily since the mucosa then lies against this abnormality smoothly and with few folds (fig. 18). We have less difficulty only when an abnormality is seen by chance in the narrow space between 2 loops which are in a more or less hypotonic phase.

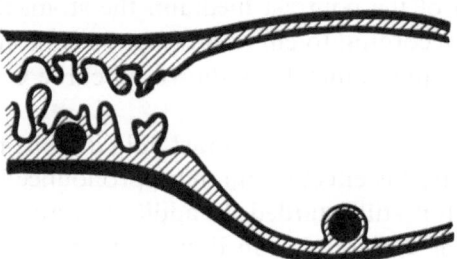

Fig. 18
An abnormality of the mucosa is more clearly visible when the intestine is in a state of dilatation than in a state of contraction.

This combination of favourable factors occurs of course only seldom.

In certain cases, if we should find it desirable, dilatation of the small intestine can be enhanced by an injection of atropine or TEAB (tetraethylammonium bromide). With atropine, the movements of the muscularis mucosa still exist, not with TEAB; the paralyzing effect of this substance is so strong that there is no motion at all (89).

After these preparations are injected, passage comes to a standstill and as a result superposition increases due to dilatation and possibly also lengthening of the loops of the small intestine. Intervention with these drugs is therefore only to be considered in the last phase of the examination after sufficient normal exposures have been made.

Theoretically it would appear sensible to restrict superposition by fractional administration of the contrast medium. The most even distribution of the contrast fluid in the small intestine is obtained by dividing the total amount into as many fractions as possible which are then administered so slowly that the continuity of the contrast column is just maintained. The contrast medium could also be administered until the cecum is reached and then a number of exposures of the entire small intestine are made. In this way, with a restricted number of photographs, the greatest amount of information could be obtained.

Just as sensible theoretically is the method of following a small amount of contrast medium to the cecum without the slightest problem of superposition. With this method, of course, exposures must be made within short time intervals which means a large radiation exposure for the patient. For each oral administration of the contrast medium, we must realize that we can regulate the supply to the stomach easily but that the passage from stomach to duodenum can only be regulated by influencing the pylorus mechanism.

Orally administered contrast medium does not leave the stomach at a constant rate, but at a gradually decreasing rate. When HENDERSON's (84) results are plotted on a graph, the resulting curve will resemble curve A in fig. 16. It shows clearly that greater gastric filling only slightly lengthens the gastric emptying time while the average rate of gastric emptying increases. It is clear that the decrease in the tone of the gastric wall and the gradual decrease in the supply of contrast medium to the pylorus cause the curve to become increasingly horizontal as the stomach becomes almost empty. We have seen that the rate of gastric emptying increases in the right lateral position. When the stomach is full, the effect is insignificant; when it is nearly empty however there is an obvious gain as a result of the considerably improved supply of contrast medium to the pylorus.

In the left lateral position of course gastric emptying will be the slowest. Some mothers learn to lay their babies on their sides after a feeding and to alternate between the right and left sides. It is not impossible that this factor plays an important role for the high average gastric emptying time determined for babies (21).

For fractional administration of the contrast medium, the stomach is only partially filled; in the ideal case, emptying will occur according to curve B of fig. 16. For equal fractions administered too rapidly, the stomach will empty approximately as shown on curve C and D of fig. 16.

Mixing proteins and carbohydrates through the contrast fluid inhibits peristalsis and keeps the pylorus closed for longer periods. For fats, this effect is still more pronounced; even 8 hours after a meal rich in fats, peristalsis of the stomach is still retarded. In addition it appeared that in healthy individuals flocculation and segmentation of the contrast medium only occurred when they had consumed a meal rich in fats the evening before (56, 178). Experiments with dogs showed that even a high or low blood sugar curve can markedly influence gastric peristalsis and the rate of transit (123). Hunger contractions when the blood sugar is low also occur in humans.

The pylorus remains closed when the contents of the stomach or duodenum are highly acidic or basic. For patients with achlorhydria this closing mechanism does not function as well; the pylorus is more relaxed and the stomach therefore empties quickly.

We also saw that isotonic solutions leave the stomach the fastest and that hypotonic solutions do not take much longer. However when a hypotonic solution is introduced directly into the duodenum the pylorus will remain closed until a condition of isotonicity is achieved (66). Hypertonic solutions retard gastric emptying considerably, even when they are administered directly into the duodenum. In the stomach, a hypertonic solution gradually becomes isotonic as a result of heavy fluid secretion of the gastric wall. This can be accompanied by a considerably increase in volume.

Cold fluids leave the stomach much faster and warm fluids only slightly slower than a solution at body temperature (65). The rapid transit of a cold fluid through the small intestine can certainly be ascribed in part to the accelerated gastric emptying. The reaction of gastric peristalsis and the pylorus to the direct administration of cold or warm fluids into the duodenum has unfortunately not yet been studied; the mechanism for this temperature sensitivity is also unknown. Furthermore it is important to know that the activating of the neutralization mechanism in the duodenum, a reaction to milieu disturbances of all kinds, does not begin until after the bulb and then decreases in the distal direction (1, 11, 66, 103, 118, 178, 190).

The contrast medium has a very difficult time during a gastro-intestinal examination; it must successively endure the influence of gastric acid, intestinal juice and fluid withdrawal without losing its proper characteristics. In some cases, there is also the detrimental effect of fatty acids, gall or lactic acid which practically no contrast medium can tolerate.

Diverse brands can withstand the effect of gastric acid and mucin reasonably well but only a few contrast media can endure dehydration without becoming practically useless. The viscosity then becomes so high that the soft mucosal folds cause few impressions, or none at all. The specific gravity of the contrast mass increases; it retains however its homogeneous structure.

We can see that the contrast medium is about to loose the battle when flocculation develops; if in addition segmentation has already developed, then it has definitely lost. The structure of these segment clumps is not homogeneous as in the case of dehydration; the genesis is also different. If it is understandable that a highly thickened contrast medium is no longer able to produce true mucosal patterns, it must then be obvious for a splotchy segment clump (fig. 34). In 1942 BOUSLOG had already seen moulage-like patterns in small children which were not in agreement with the normal mucosal patterns seen at autopsy; the reason for this incongruity was then not understood.

If we study the curves of BRAECKMAN and ZIMMER, we learn that disintegration of the contrast medium is a physicochemical process which proceeds gradually and that even in the most unfavourable circumstances we still have a few minutes to make a number of useful roentgenograms. Fig. 51 shows the results which can be obtained even with a very thin contrast medium of moderate stability, in a patient with a severe fatty diarrhea.

From the preceding it can be seen that it is sensible to give large amounts of contrast medium; the influence of harmful substances on the contrast medium is then less. Furthermore it is obvious that this dosage must pass through the small intestine as rapidly as possible; reaction with the harmful substances is then short-lived and the detrimental effect is as small as possible.

Another important advantage of an extremely rapid passage is the lack of time for dehydration of the contrast medium in the distal ileum and the colon. Because the low viscosity is maintained, mucosal patterns with a maximum reproduction of detail can also be obtained for these sections of the distal intestine. It is not easy to choose among the large number of brands of contrast medium on the market. There are some which are reasonably satisfactory but no single brand can be called ideal.

In 1932, ADAM (2) had already reported that the characteristics of the contrast medium suspension are determined predominantly by chemical additives and not the particle size, as is so often suggested by the manufacturers. The requirements for a contrast medium used for a gastro-intestinal examination are much higher than for a colon examination. For the latter good adhesion to the mucosa is of decisive importance; for the former, sufficient stability to prevent flocculation is of even greater importance. Furthermore the viscosity may not be too high and must be maintained in so far as possible under the influence of fluid withdrawal in the ileum.

Supplementary administration of cooled fluids and fluid attracting or secretion enhancing substances is strongly discouraged. Mixture of glucose, Gastrografine or Sorbitol with the contrast fluid has an unfavourable effect in this respect. It is difficult to determine with certainty whether or not prostigmin and metoclopramide are completely free of a secretion enhancing effect.

Summarizing it must be concluded that a large quantity of contrast medium should be administered by infusion directly into the duodenum. It should be administered so quickly that the stretching of the duodenum induces maximum peristalsis, but not so quickly that peristalsis is inhibited by the entero-intestinal reflex mechanism or that the patient will vomit. The amount of contrast medium must be as large as possible but then again not so large that the problem of superposition develops.

The contrast fluid must be hypotonic; hypertonia stimulates fluid attraction and therefore dilution of the contrast fluid; isotonia does not stimulate contraction of the pyloric muscle and in this way enhances the development of reflux into the stomach.

Another advantage of by-passing the stomach is that the detrimental effect of gastric acid on the contrast fluid is eliminated and that the rate of supply to the duodenum is no longer dependent upon the pyloric function.

Since most brands are reasonably stable in alkaline surroundings, we are less restricted now in the choice of contrast medium; the adhesive quality and the viscosity can be the decisive factors. From the above it will be clear that the unrealized ideal of standardization of the contrast medium, desired by so many radiologists has as a result of this method outlived itself. A continuous supply of contrast fluid without the annoying influence of air bubbles, which possibly also retard transit, is only guaranteed in the right lateral position. The patient may possibly also lie on his back or on his abdomen but in any event, the left lateral position is incorrect.

The question of the most favourable temperature for the contrast medium will not be considered further in this study; it requires further investigation.

It is true that an ice-cold contrast fluid does enhance gastric emptying and intestinal peristalsis but when administered into the duodenum, possibly also relaxation of the pylorus so that reflux into the stomach could occur. A warm contrast fluid keeps the pylorus closed longer but could even work as a transit decelerator when administered directly into the duodenum. For our examinations therefore a relatively neutral standpoint is taken; all patients received the contrast medium at room temperature

(20–22 °C). Also unanswered is the question of the most favourable location for the end of the tube in the duodenum. It is possible that reflux into the stomach is more likely when the end of the tube lies proximal; then when the contrast fluid is administered, maximum stretching of the duodenum occurs quite close to the pylorus which as a result may not close as well.

Another factor is the pyloric muscle which is usually relaxed; it takes several seconds before contraction occurs. It is clear that at least some reflux of contrast fluid into the stomach will occur when the end of the tube lies close to the open pyloric canal.

Thirdly a tube located in the proximal part of the duodenum can slip back into the stomach as a result of regurgitation.

On the basis of these somewhat speculative considerations, in our patients the end of the tube was placed in the duodeno-jejunal area, although it must be assumed that the peristalsis induced by stretching of the intestinal wall is less here than close to the bulb.

It is possible that in achlorhydria reflux of the contrast fluid into the stomach will occur sooner; this question cannot be answered and requires further study. As mentioned previously it is obvious that reflux cannot be terminated once it has occurred. The best thing to do is a supplementary dosage of contrast medium administered at once as well as stimulation of gastric emptying with Primperan. Obviously the patient must lie on the right lateral side between exposures.

In all cases we must concentrate on 'forcing' the contrast medium to the cecum as quickly as possible. Especially in patients with a possible malabsorption syndrome, the disintegration of the contrast medium can occur so quickly that examination of the small intestine must be considered a 'case of great haste'.

VIII
THE ENTERAL CONTRAST INFUSION

Preparation of patients

Even more important than for a conventional follow-through study is the thorough cleansing of the patient; it is even desirable that the stomach be entirely empty and thus contain no fasting gastric residuum. Should there be gastric fluid in the stomach, the pylorus will not close properly since it is a natural reaction of the stomach to dispel its contents through the pyloric canal. When an infusion is running, the pressure in the duodenum is probably greater than the pressure in the stomach so that the open pyloric canal will have a reverse effect on gastric emptying and reflux of the contrast fluid into the stomach from the duodenum will occur.

The day before the examination the diet must be a low residue diet and the last meal preferably free of fats.

Since it is possible that the presence of feces in the cecum can retard passage, it is also advisable to give the patient a laxative. If the cecum is thoroughly cleansed, very good exposures can generally be made which are not inferior to those from a conventional colon examination. Before the examination we used to give the patient an enema, but sometimes such a reflux of the cecum contents into the ileum occurred that this is no longer a routine procedure; it is now only used when the colon films are more important than the exposures of the small intestine.

It is desirable that the patient receive no medication which inhibits the intestinal peristalsis; stimulation of gall production or contraction of the gall bladder must also be avoided.

Duodenal intubation

Probably inspired by Seldinger's catheter for vascular examination, BILBAO et al. developed a set for use in hypotonic duodenography which is similar and has highly simplified duodenal intubation. It consists of a radiopaque flexible tube with an inner diameter of 3 mm, which can carry a thick metal feed line. The tube is slightly less pliable than a normal duodenal tube of the same diameter; on the proximal end is a luer-lock adapter. The distal end is closed but just inside are a number of openings in the wall of the tube.

The metal feed line has a diameter of 1.5 mm and is derived from the rotating inner cable of the Volkswagon speedometer. The outer spiral wires of this cable have been removed so that the inner spiral layer and a number of centrally located longitudinal steel wires are left over. The Volkswagen adapter is removed from one end of the cable and the wires are soldered together with silver.

The Bilbao set is very expensive; it is however simple to make such a set which is highly satisfactory and does not cost one-tenth the price. A normal radiopaque duodenal tube is quite suitable. On the distal end is a metal olive-shaped bead with holes or grooves only in the wall. As feed line, a Volkswagon speedometer cable can indeed be used. It costs a half hour to remove the outer spiral layer from the inner cable and to solder a silver tip on one end. If desired, the feed line of the Bilbao tube can also be purchased separately.

A disadvantage of the Bilbao tube is that the feed line can very easily be slid through one of the openings of the tube (fig. 19). If the last part of the procedure is not carried out under fluoroscopic

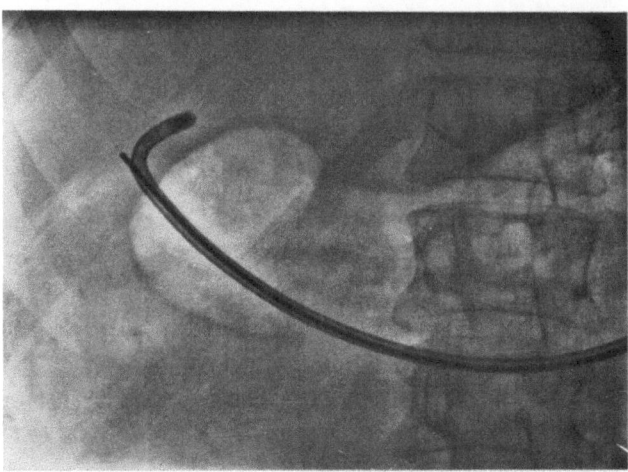

Fig. 19
Feed line extends through side openings in the old model of the Bilbao-Dotter tube (danger of perforations and mucosal lesions). With the new Bilbao-Dotter tube, which is longer than the old one, this can no longer occur since the tube is longer than the feed line.

control, it could easily lead to damage to the mucosa and even perforation of the gastric wall. If the tube has an olive-shaped metal end, the risk does not exist as long as there is no opening at the end or this opening is so small that the silver tip of the feed line cannot pass through.

A second disadvantage of the Bilbao tube is that when the stomach is located high in the abdomen, it is not always possible to slide the moderately flexible tube in the antral direction; the tube then keeps curling up in the pars cardiaca. Because of the resulting tight loops, it is not possible to slide the stiff metal feed line through the tube. It is of course senseless to intubate the tube with the feed line in it; furthermore this increases the risk of perforation. This difficulty only arose for a few patients, but it was then always possible to introduce the more pliable Rehfuss tube. When the patient lies on his right side and leans slightly forward, the tube will keep falling in the direction of the pylorus due to the weight of the metal end.

Introduction of the tube only costs several minutes when one proceeds as follows. The patient swallows the tube while standing or sitting. When it passes the larynx, a choking reflex develops which only lasts a short time if the tube is quickly pushed in further. Some patients and doctors prefer to introduce the tube through the nasal cavity instead of orally, but this is not to be advised since manipulation of the feed line can then be exceedingly difficult.

The tube is pushed on until the metal end is approximately in the pars pylorica of the stomach. The patient is then placed on his back for fluoroscopic control. If it appears that the tube curls or bends sharply, then it must be pulled back into the pars media and sometimes even into the pars cardiaca. If the stomach contains too much fasting residuum, it is desirable to wait until it has disappeared through the tube. The metal feed line is now pushed through the tube; this is easier when the patient opens his mouth and bends his head as far back as possible.

It is very important that the feed line not be pushed all the way to the end of the tube but that the last 5–10 cm remain flexible; this greatly increases the ease and safety of the procedure since only the flexible tube passes through the pyloric canal. For very large, ptotic stomachs, it is sometimes even necessary that the last 20 cm of the tube remain flexible.

The combination is now pushed further in the direction of the duodenum under fluoroscopic control; this is easier when the patient lies on his right side. The stiffness of the feed line prevents curling of the tube in the stomach. When the end of the tube appears to move in the direction of the spinal column and then slightly downwards, it is practically certain that the pyloric canal has been passed. It is exceptional for the pyloric canal to deviate from this direction. Sometimes the pyloric muscle is slightly spastic or a vomiting reflex occurs as a result of manipulation with the tube; we have found that patience is the quickest way to success. The end of the tube must be pushed forward to the distal part of the duodenum; it is very important that the feed line be pulled back each time so that it does not pass the pyloric canal. Not until the tube is in the correct position is the feed line removed. Should the feed line enter the duodenum anyway, then it is curled so much that it is usually no longer possible to remove it. The whole combination must then first be pulled back into the stomach.

It is superfluous to mention that only a moderate fluoroscopic current (for BV–TV 0.5–1 mA) is necessary for this procedure and that the field need not be greater than 50 cm².

Due to various causes (psyche, steer-horn stomach, severe ptosis, pyloric spasm, constrictions, etc.) the introduction of the tube can take a little longer for some patients; however this need not often exceed 10 minutes. It is obvious that experience plays an important role; in the beginning, we did not succeed in the intubation of 2 patients at all.

Administration of the contrast medium

This phase of the examination determines the quality of the mucosal patterns obtained; diverse factors are responsible. After this only a good examination technique and enough exposures for each intestinal section to be seen clearly can influence the information obtained.

Although it would seem obvious that the contrast medium chosen is probably the most important factor for the success of the examination, it turns out that this is not true. If, according to the curves of BRAECKMAN and ZIMMER, the cecum is reached within 5 minutes then the results obtained with the various brands of contrast media will differ only slightly. The stability of the contrast medium, the most important characteristic for a conventional examination, plays only a secondary role in an infusion technique which is carried out correctly. The contrast media which excel in this respect, such as Mixobar and especially Raybar, do not therefore come into their own with this examination technique; in addition, Mixobar was too viscous for the required specific gravity and had therefore already been eliminated for this reason. Another characteristic of the contrast fluid which decreases in importance as the rate of transit increases is the ability to remain thin and liquid in the ileum.

The best mucosal patterns were obtained with Micropaque, but an unfortunate disadvantage of this medium is that not only in vitro but also in vivo small gas bubbles are easilyfor med (fig. 67). The viscosity of Micropaque increases quite a lot during dehydration but if we keep the transit time short, this need not cause any trouble.

Our purpose therefore is to administer the smallest amount of contrast medium without reflux into the stomach so fast that it reaches the cecum within 5 minutes after the infusion is started. We have found that this can be achieved in most patients when 600 ml contrast medium is administered in 5 to 6 minutes in the right lateral position. A shorter period of flow could cause reflux into the stomach; a longer period of flow, as in our first patients, appeared to cause a longer transit time.

The distribution of the contrast medium over the entire small intestine is so even (figs. 20,21) that superposition occurs only seldom.

According to tests carried out in vitro the specific gravity of the contrast fluid must be 1.2–1.25 (p. 31–40). We have found that this specific gravity is indeed better than a specific gravity of 1.25–1.35 which was also used for a large number of patients.

We determined the viscosity of several contrast media using a method which suited our purposes. We let 600 ml of these contrast fluids at a temperature of 20° C run through the 2 infusion systems (Bilbao tube and Rehfuss tube) and measured the flow time for a difference in level of 2 m. The results were as follows:

Brand contrast medium: water		Specific gravity	Duration in minutes	
			Bilbao tube	Rehfuss tube
Bario-dif	1:1	1.23	1½	3½
Micropaque	1:1	1.38	2	4¼
	2:3	1.30	1½	3½
	1:2	1.26	1¼	3
Micr. AZL		1.32	1	2½
Mixobar	1:3	1.2	3½	10½
	1:2	1.28	10½	—

The viscosity of the Mixobar appeared to be so high that this medium must be considered less suited for this examination method with our infusion systems. Although extensive experiments are required to justify the choice of a brand of contrast medium, we tentatively chose Micropaque on the basis of the impressions received.

Because passage of the contrast medium through the small intestine is already very rapid, it is senseless to use accelerating drugs. That Bario-dif already contains Sorbitol is therefore considered a disadvantage. The limited value of metoclopramide (Primperan) for this examination technique was very nicely demonstrated in several patients from the initial stages of our study. Because at that time the infusion still lasted 10 minutes or more, the cecum had sometimes not yet been reached even after 20 minutes. It appeared that an intravenous injection of 20 mg Primperan caused a short period of more active peristalsis of the small intestine; but it apparently had little effect since usually the cecum had still not been reached 10 minutes later. On the other hand however when a supplementary 300–600 ml contrast medium was administered, a more active peristalsis also developed and by the end of the infusion, the cecum had indeed been reached. As a result of these experiences, it is now routine procedure to give a second dosage of contrast medium if the cecum has not been reached 5 minutes after the end of the first infusion. It is striking that even with this large amount of contrast medium, superposition is so slight that it cannot be used as an argument against the procedure described (figs. 21, 54, 56). Because a certain intestinal segment had to be examined in more detail, we were fortunate enough to be able to administer a contrast infusion with and one without 20 mg Primperan to one patient five days apart under otherwise equal conditions. As was expected, there was no difference in the rate of transit at all.

Although therefore metoclopramide apparently has a separate effect on the peristalsis of the small intestine, the transit acceleration caused by this substance during an oral examination must be ascribed predominantly to the accelerated gastric emptying and not a more active peristalsis of the small intestine.

After the infusion, the tube is not removed but is washed clean with 20 ml water and then closed with a cap.

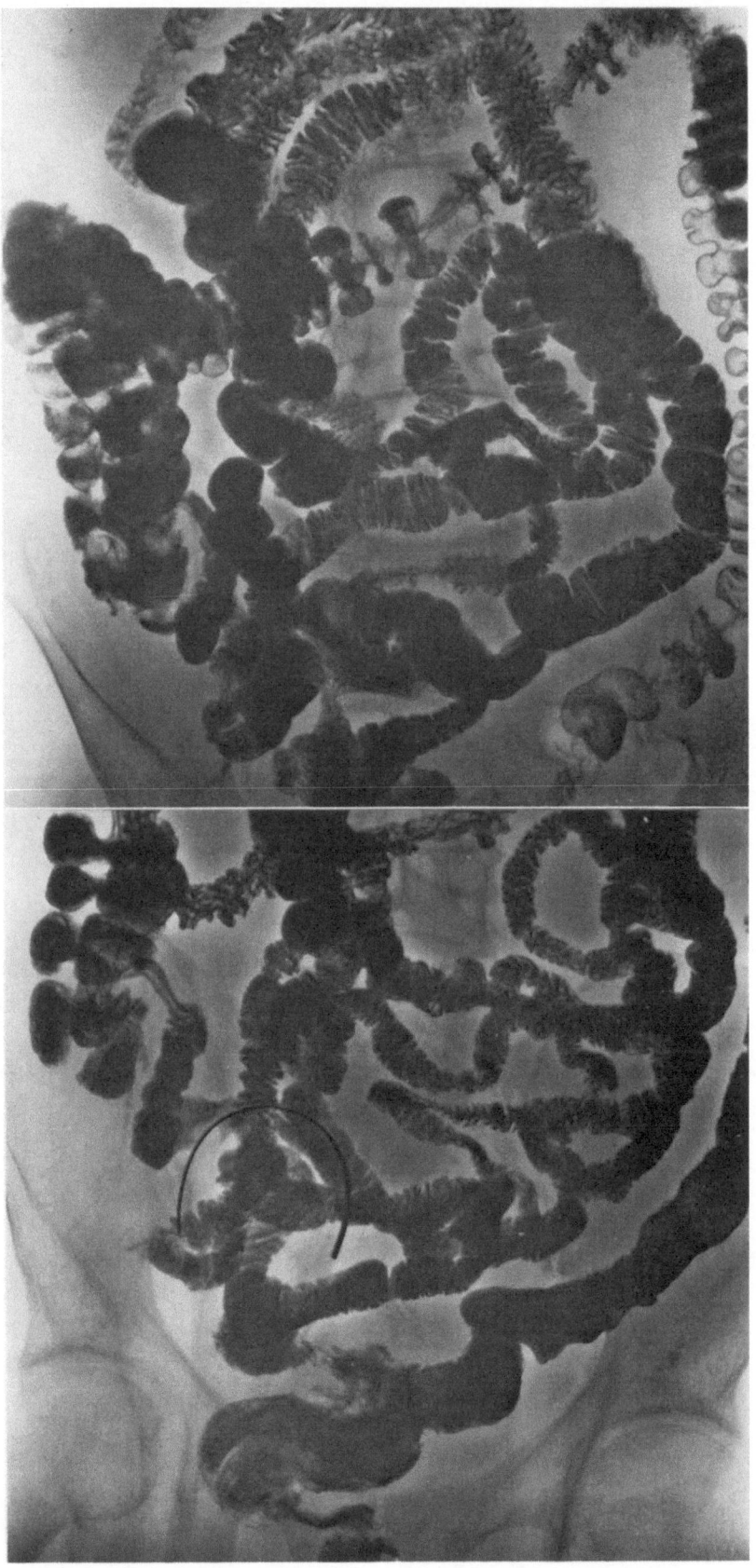

Fig. 20
Especially for pycnics, the position of
the loops of the small intestine is
usually quite clear. Filling with 600 ml
contrast fluid.

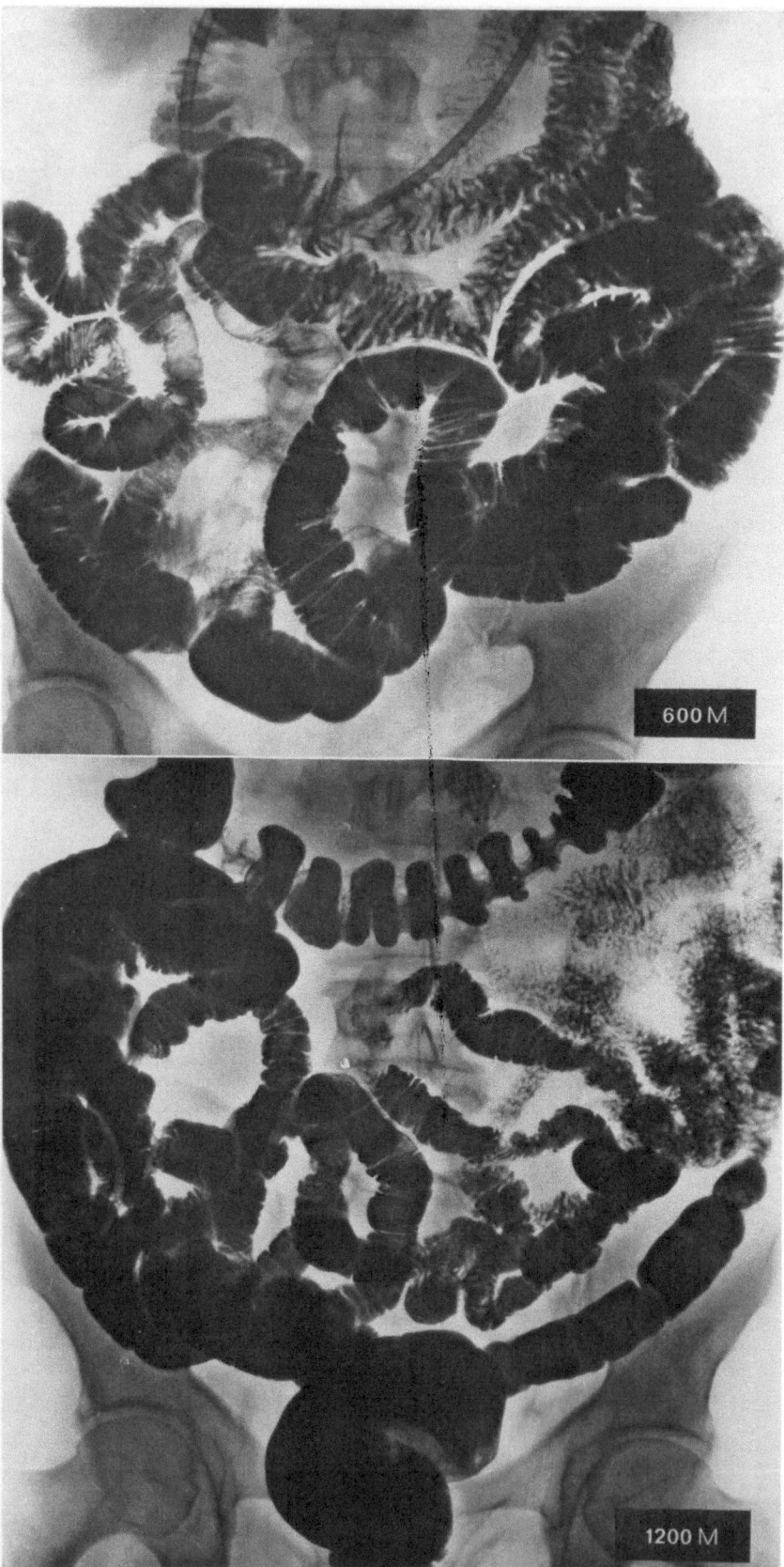

Fig. 21
Status after ileo-cecal resection
because of Crohn's disease. Clear
picture, even after administration
of 1200 ml contrast fluid.

Radiological examination

To obtain the best possible roentgenological examination of the small intestine, it is vitally important that the instructions given for the administration of the contrast infusion be followed exactly. Although it is always possible that the technique will be improved, every variation so far has resulted in inferior exposures. It is therefore advisable to compare the results of a proposed change with those of the technique described here.

At the end of the infusion period, which lasts 4 to 5 minutes, the loops of the duodenum, jejunum and ileum are usually filled with contrast fluid. In a number of cases it will still take a few minutes for the cecum to be reached.

If reflux into the stomach has occurred, the examination will usually last considerably longer (p. 87). In such cases, it has been found that an immediate supplementary dosage of contrast medium is useful and that the dosage should increase as the amount of contrast fluid flowing back into the stomach increases. Some of this second dosage will of course again end up in the stomach. Under fluoroscopic control, care should be taken that the stomach is not filled too full because when this occurs the patient will vomit both the gastric contents and the tube. We usually add 15 ml Primperan to this supplementary dosage in the hope that gastric emptying will be enhanced to the greatest possible degree.

We have already seen that an extra 300–600 ml contrast medium is also administered if the cecum has not yet been reached 5 or 6 minutes after termination of the first contrast fluid infusion. If no reflux into the stomach has occurred, it is useless to add Primperan.

In cases of malabsorption, the contrast fluid is more likely to flocculate; the first part of the Braeckman curve will therefore be steeper. It is obvious that for these patients a second contrast medium dosage should be considered immediately if the cecum has not yet been reached, instead of waiting 5 or 6 minutes. The stability of the contrast medium used will also play a role in this decision; Raybar for instance will not flocculate as quickly and in the case of malabsorption, the Braeckman curve will be considerably less steep for Raybar than for Microbar AZL.

It is recommended that during the infusion period 2 exposures be made showing the jejunal loops clearly without the interference of superimposed ileum loops filled with contrast medium. At the end of the contrast infusion, survey exposures are made while the patient is lying on his abdomen; now the entire jejunum and ileum are usually seen. It is wise to make series of 2 or 3 exposures; as a result of the small time intervals, the intestinal loops are then seen in the same position but often in different phases of contraction.

Then under fluoroscopic control with a field of 100 of 200 cm^2, the entire small intestine is studied for eventual abnormalities. It must be emphasized that this is an essential part of the examination as pointed out by GOOD (77) and many other investigators (78, 221). In general, examination of the ileum loops and the ileocecal area will require the most time. There are more abnormalities which can be diagnosed by the radiologist in the ileum than in the equally long jejunum; in addition free projection of the ileum loops is more difficult.

It is obvious that compression is indispensible in this phase of the examination. We have learned that the large flat compressors of the modern tele-command roentgen apparatus are much more satisfactory for free projection of larger intestinal segments than the spoon of Holzknecht, which is only suitable for highly circumscribed lesions. This led us to construct a large compressor, using the inner ball of a soccer ball mounted on a plastic pipe, for conventional roentgen apparatus. Fig. 22 shows the construction of this spoon which is quite satisfactory in practice.

Another advantage of the modern roentgen apparatus is that a craniad or caudalward beam direction can be chosen which makes an angle of 0° to 30° with the conventional vertical central beam.

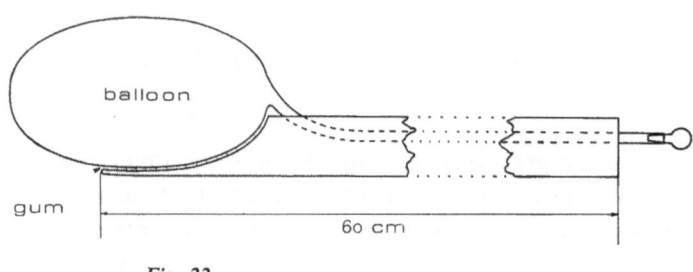

Fig. 22
Home-made hand-compressor

It must be mentioned that relatively little use is made of this for the examination of the small intestine since the quality of the pictures is visibly better with a vertical beam and in addition the more important compression is carried out more efficiently.

A third advantage of this apparatus is that under fluoroscopic control exposures of the small intestine can be made while the patient lies on his abdomen which clearly show less geometrical vagueness than those made under conventional conditions because of the more favourable projection ratios.

Even in the abdominal position it is not always possible to get the ileum loops out of the small pelvis. In such cases we have found that it can be advantageous to place the patient in a Trendelenburg position, sometimes even up to 45°, for several minutes. The use of shoulder supports is of course indispensible for these manipulations. The barium-filled, heavier ileum loops slip slowly out of the small pelvis against the abdominal wall so that useful survey exposures can be made.

The total amount of time for examination and exposures is usually 10 to 15 minutes, sometimes less, sometimes much more. For some patients, passage is so rapid that even the entire colon and rectosigmoid can become filled in 5 to 10 minutes. It is understandable that examination of the ileum can be exceedingly difficult in this situation. It is therefore necessary to work quickly and not waste time. For our first patients, fluoroscopy lasted 15 to 20 minutes (90 kV, 0.3–1 mA), but after some practice it will appear that more than 10 minutes is seldom necessary. During the entire examination the fluoroscopic field may not be larger than absolutely necessary.

For various reasons, it might be useful in some cases to expand the examination by using special techniques which shall now be discussed.

Supplementary administration of air or water

It seems justified to discuss this technique separately and, for the time being, not to regard it as an integral part of the examination of the small intestine.

During the colon examination, pea-sized defects can be missed completely on the filling or mucosal exposures. Double-contrast exposures have appeared to be such a valuable supplement that they have become almost a necessary part of the colon examination. The diameter of the loops of the small intestine is however so much smaller that pea-sized filling defects in the contrast medium are not as easily missed when sufficient exposure is used.

In addition, in the small intestine superposition can occasionally occur on the double-contrast exposures to such a degree that it is difficult to eliminate by compression; this seldom happens in the colon. On the other hand it must be mentioned that during an examination of the small intestine, air insufflation through the tube is sometimes the only way to get the ileum loops out of the small pelvis when the patient is lying on his back so that compression can be applied (figs. 23, 52b–c).

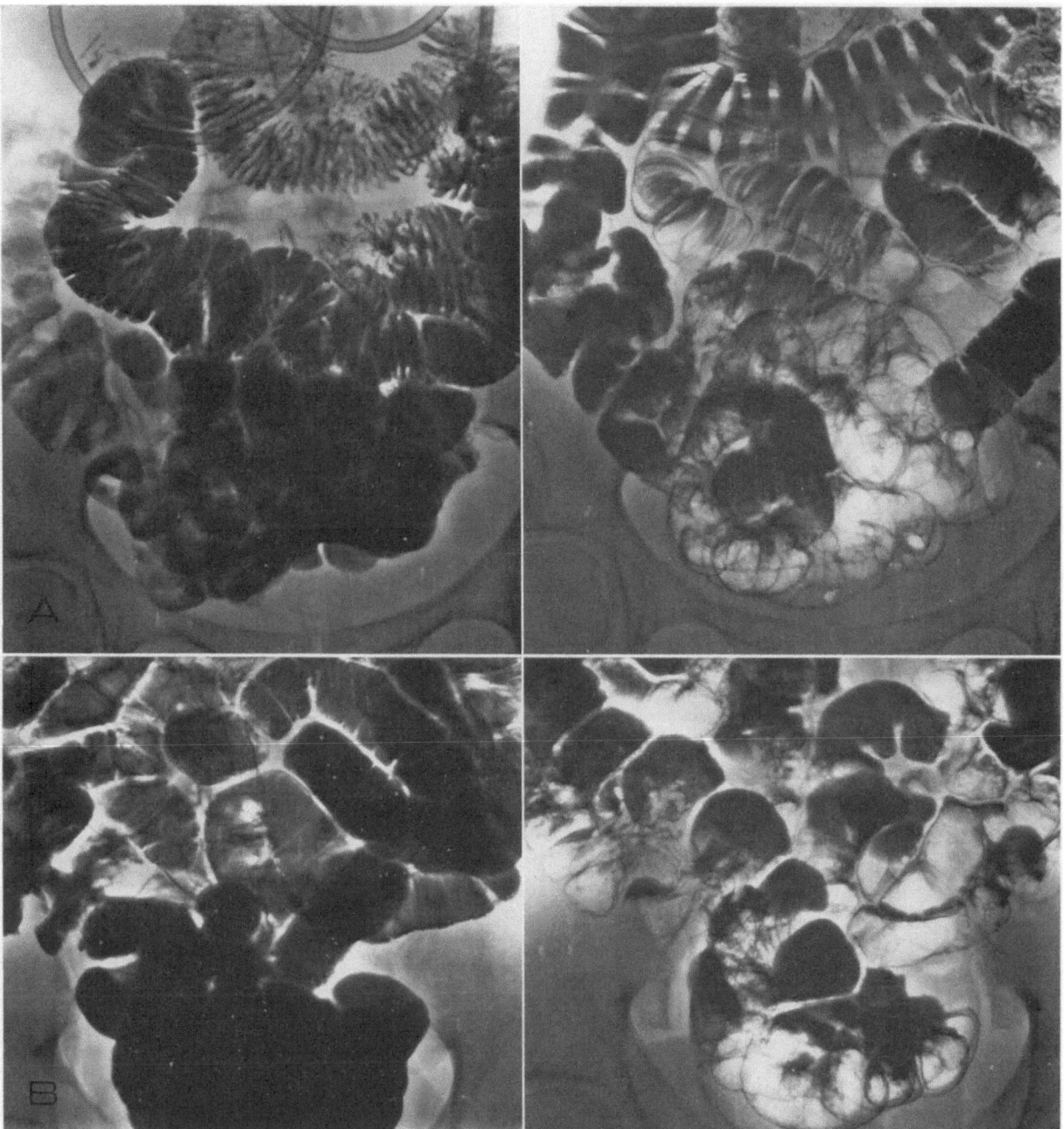

Fig. 23
Oral air insufflation in 2 patients with troublesome mass of ileum loops in small pelvis.

For oral air insufflation, a balloon or syringe sends air through the tube at regular intervals to a total of approximately 500 ml. If the air is supplied too quickly, painful abdominal cramps can occur; a dose of 200 ml per minute is easily tolerated. The air moves rapidly and independently of the contrast medium toward the cecum. In this way, outstanding exposures of the entire small intestine and even the colon can often be obtained (figs. 24, 25 and 26). Peristaltic waves are so intense that sometimes local blurring due to movement is observed on the roentgenogram.

Long after air insufflation, filling pictures can still be obtained of the small intestine but they are

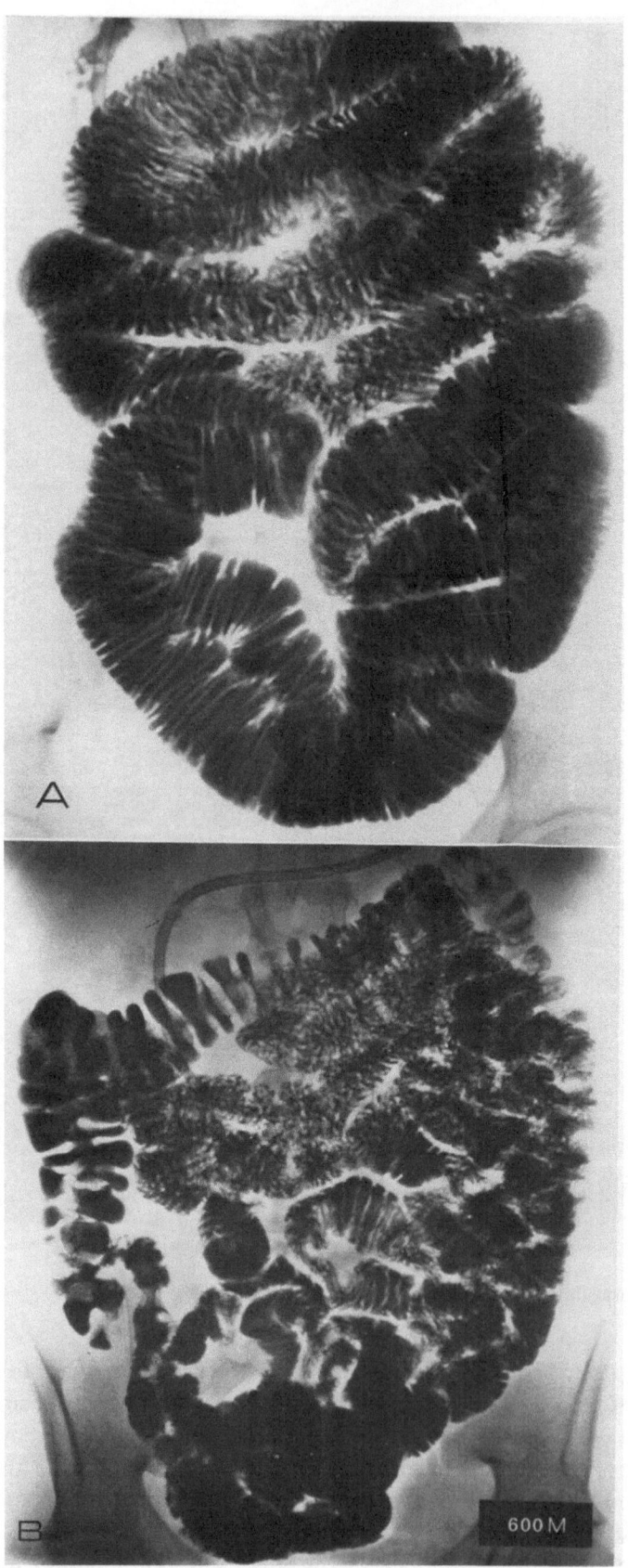

Fig. 24
Standard examination with oral air insufflation
A: during contrast medium infusion.
B: at the end of the infusion.

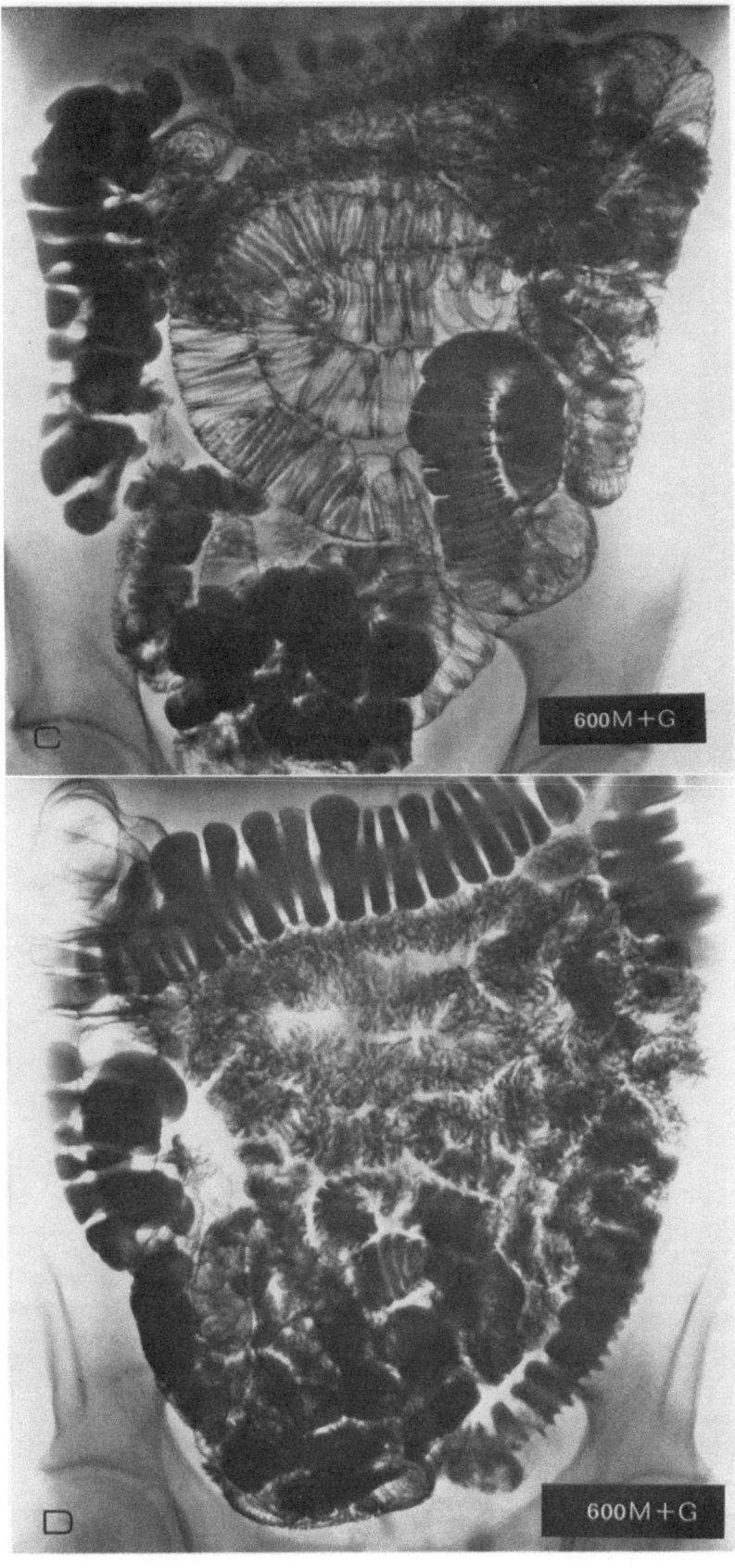

Fig. 24
c: air administered through tube is.
   seen in jejunum
d: air is located in ileum and colon.

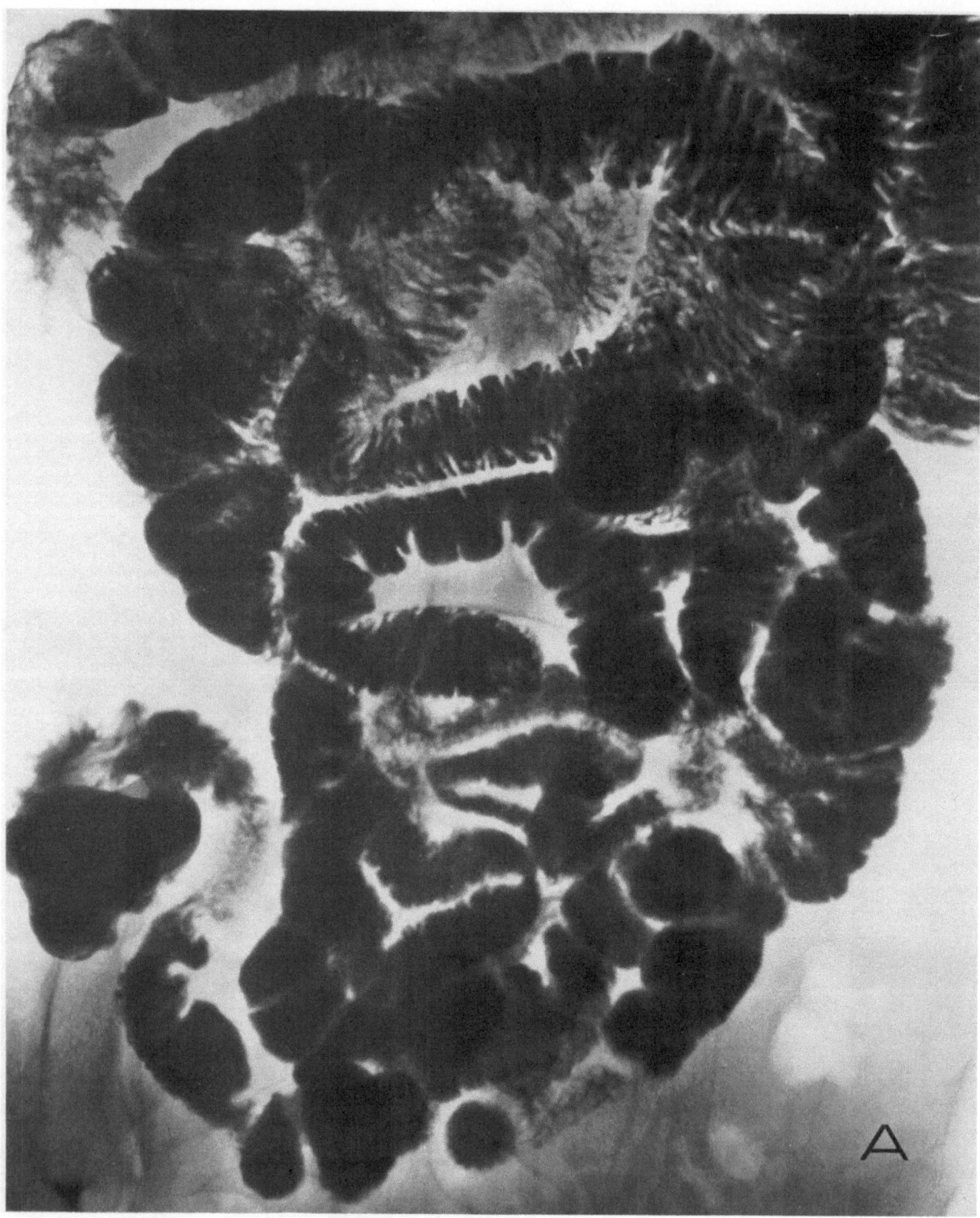

Fig. 25
A: Exposure at the end of infusion of 600 ml contrast medium.

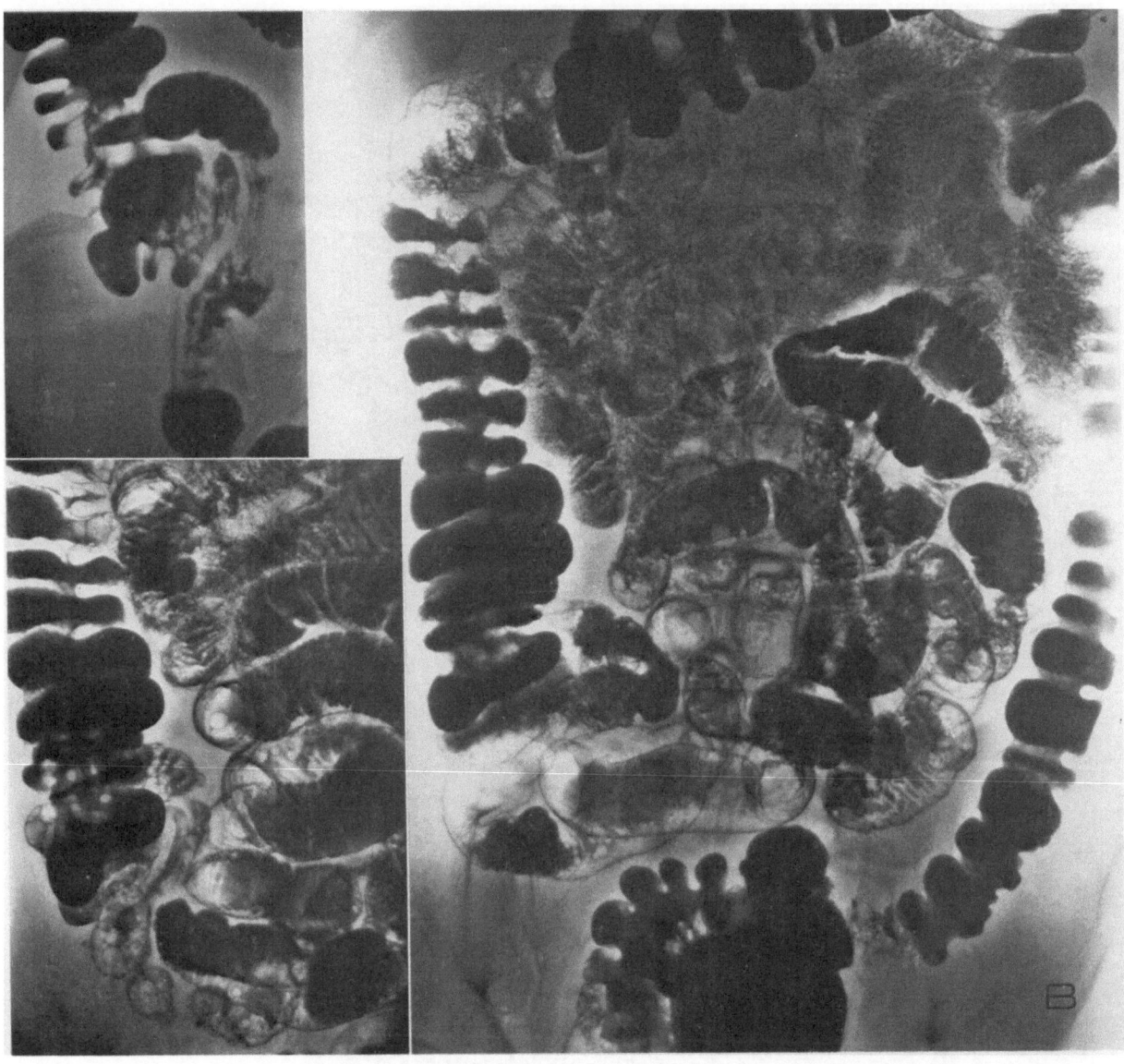

Fig. 25
B: air in ileum and colon after insufflation through tube.

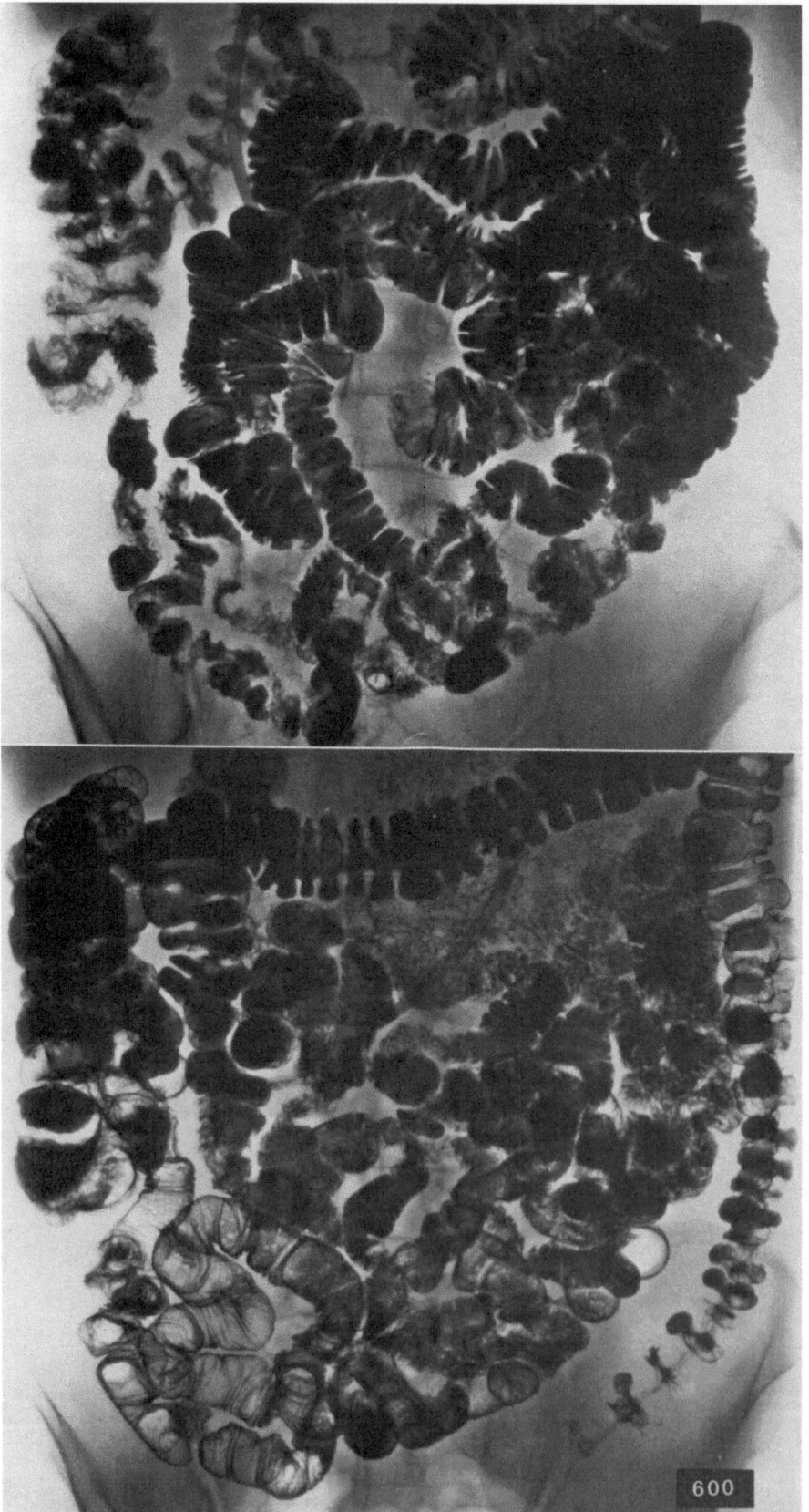

Fig. 26
A: survey exposures before
and after air insufflation
through tube.

very poor; the air is now located predominantly in the colon (fig. 27). It is remarkable that in spite of the intense peristalsis, the contrast medium barely moves during the passage of air. Should contrast filling of the rectosigmoid occur during a very rapid transit, then rectal air insufflation can sometimes be the answer, especially in the abdominal position or the Trendelenburg position; the contrast is then forced out of these sections of the intestine and in addition the ileum loops are forced out of the small pelvis (fig. 28).

Fig. 26
B: survey exposure after air insufflation through tube.

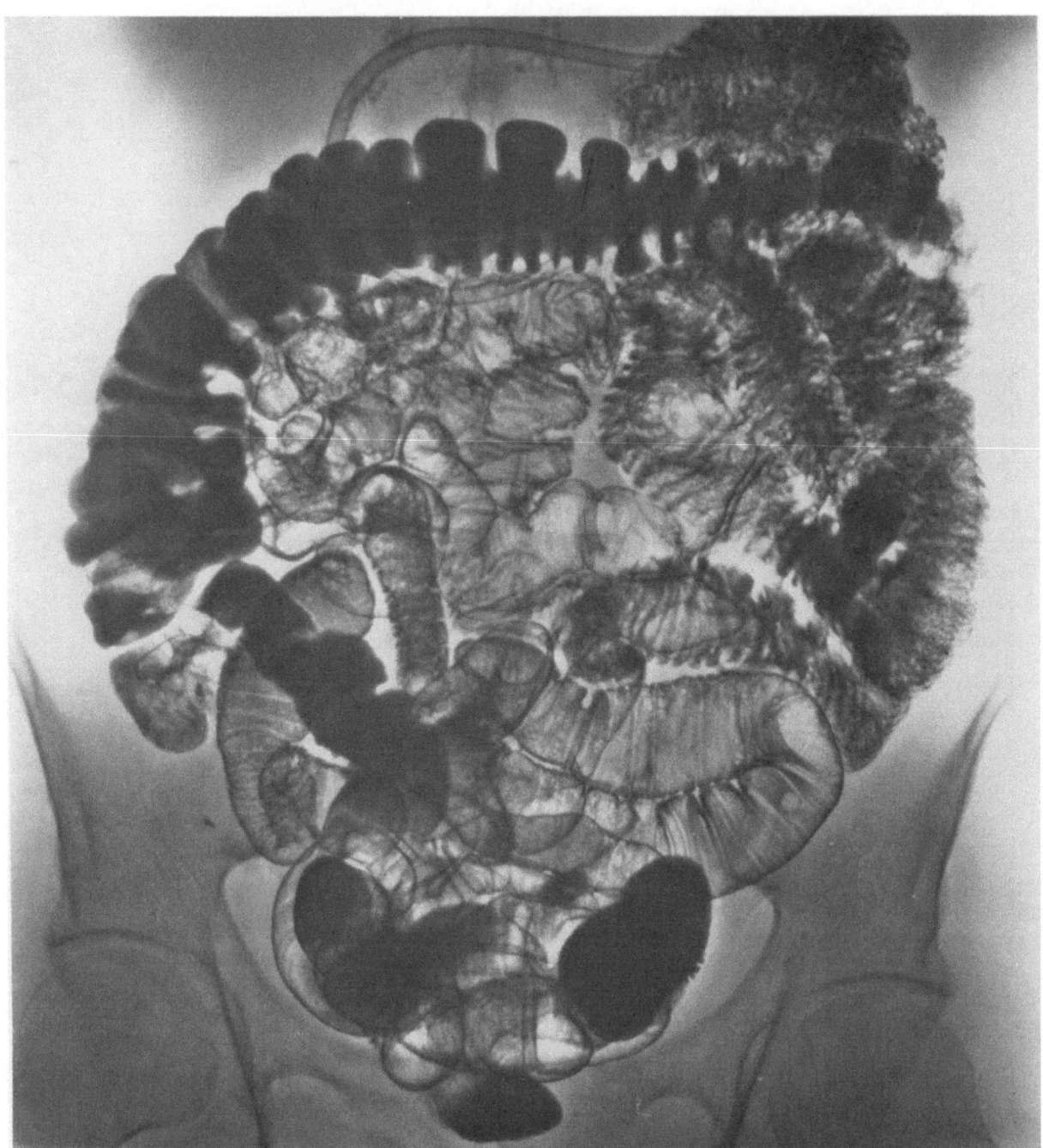

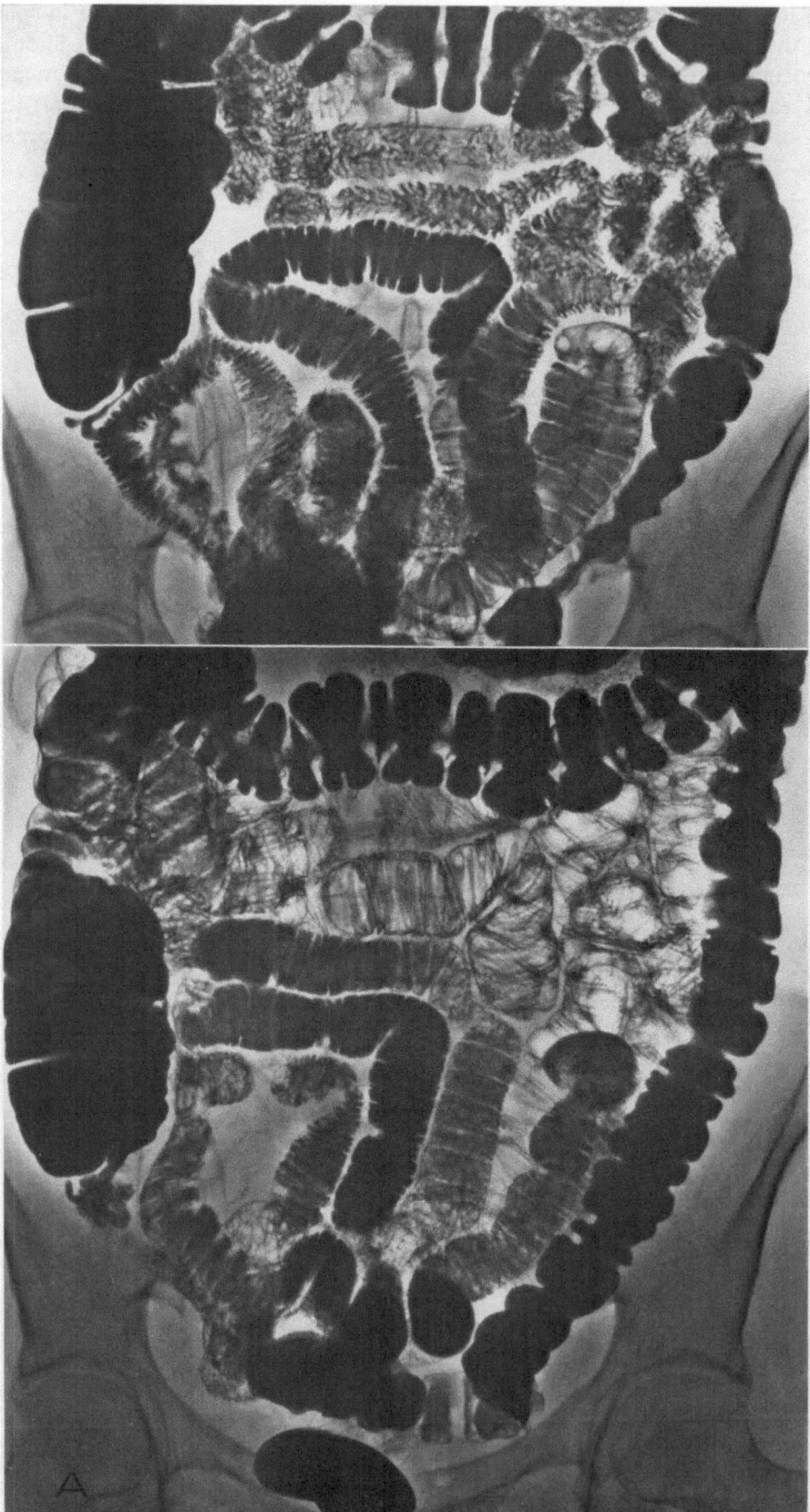

Fig. 27
A: 800 ml Microbar AZL
(s.g. 1.32) + air insufflation
through tube.

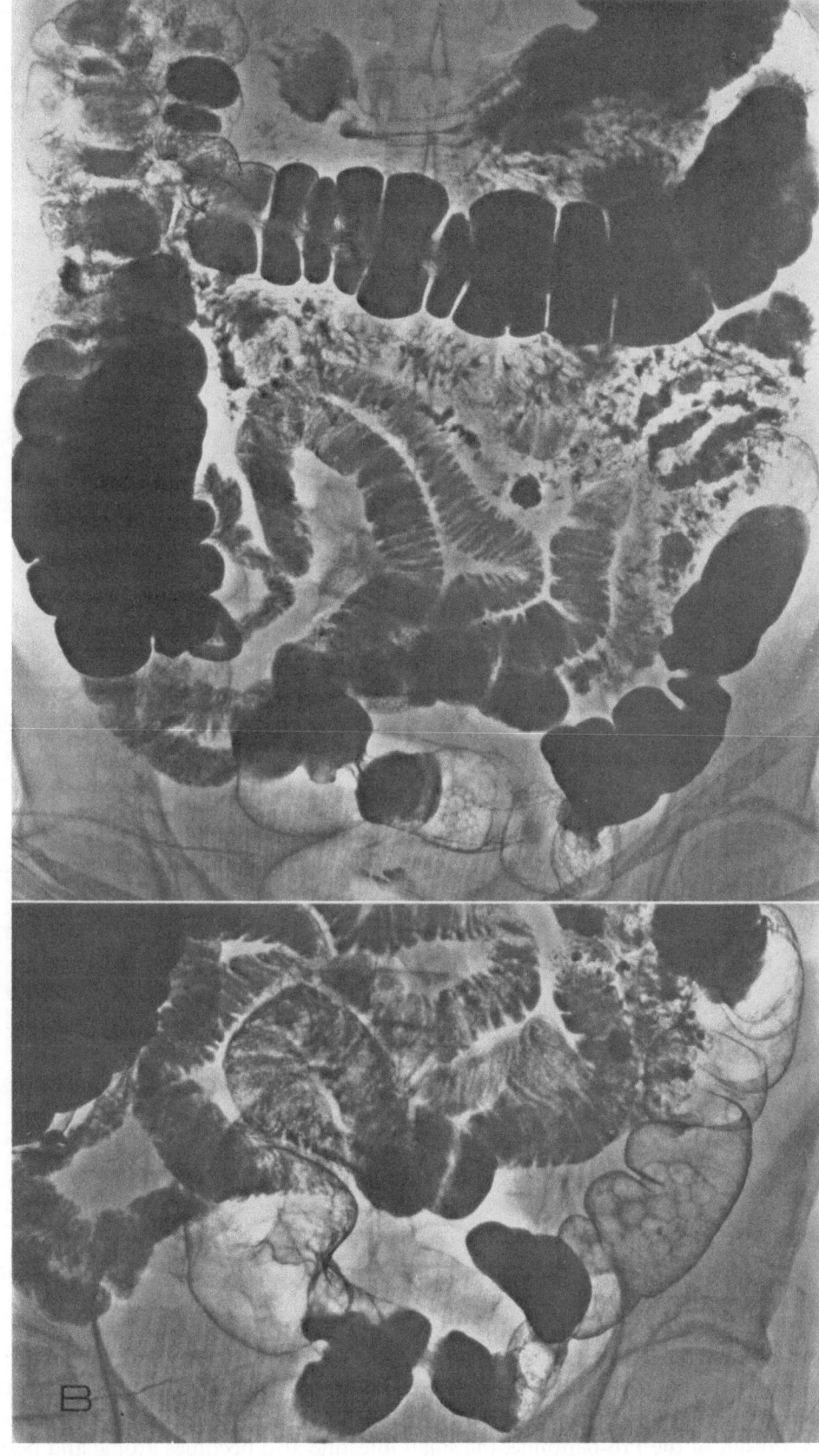

Fig. 27
B: one hour later, air
  can no longer be
  seen in the small
  intestine.
  Disintegration of
  contrast fluid in
  the jejunum.

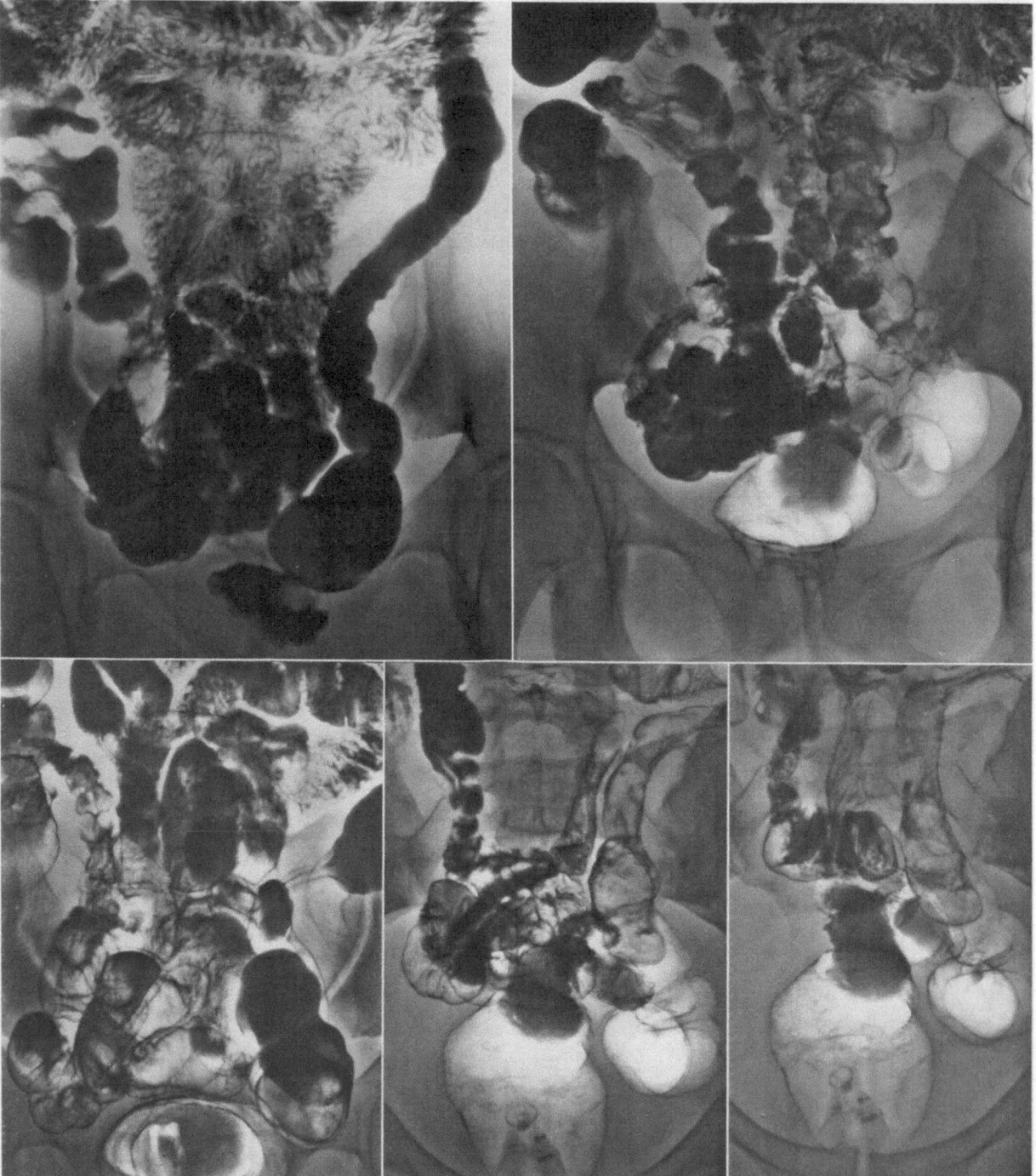

Fig. 28
Colon and ileum filled with air by rectal insufflation. Ileum loops forced out of small pelvis by means of compression.

PAJEWSKI et al. (158) recently reported a double-contrast examination of the small intestine in combination with a conventional gastro-intestinal examination. Air is introduced through a gastric tube after Pro-banthine is given to induce relaxation of the pylorus for easier passage of the air. Of course as a result of the Pro-banthine, the small intestine also becomes atonic and peristalsis is inhibited. In general only the jejunum can be shown in this manner; the distal ileum is often not even reached. Due to the increased content of the small intestinal lumen, superposition will be greater, especially when a large section is filled with air.

The contrast caused by air can sometimes be so annoying that we investigated the double-contrast technique using water in a number of patients; CUMMACK (39) uses this method regularly for the colon examination. At the end of the small bowel study, we therefore introduced 600 ml water at 18–20 °C through the tube. As in the case of the contrast infusion, the water must also be administered in 5 minutes. Since the viscosity of water is less than that of the contrast medium, the bag of water must be suspended much lower. With our infusion system it then hangs approximately 50 cm above the surface of the table. The exposures obtained in this way can also be exceptional, possibly even better than with air insufflation (figs. 29A, 29B 30).

We noticed that the barium is quickly washed off the intestinal mucosa by the water infusion and that the time available for making roentgenograms is therefore very short. It is however not at all certain that these supplementary exposures lead to an actual increase in information; this will have to be studied further in the future. It will be clear that a double-contrast examination with air, and especially with water, requires a contrast medium which adheres readily to the mucosa. Contrast fluids with a low viscosity are easily washed off the intestinal wall or leave only a thin adhesive layer. This thin layer will only be visible when the contrast fluid has a high specific gravity. In general therefore it can be stated that a low viscosity and a low specific gravity of the contrast fluid are unfavourable factors for this technique. Fig. 29A and fig. 29B show that the adhesive layer of Microbar AZL is much thinner than that of Micropaque in the concentrations we use. The higher specific gravity of Microbar AZL is not sufficient compensation for the thinness of the layer; therefore the quality of the resulting double-contrast exposures is inferior especially in comparison with the Micropaque exposures. The thickness of the adhesive layer is of course partly a question of personal taste.

It is usually not the need for double-contrast exposures which dictates a water infusion but the necessity of administering more than 1200 ml fluid while avoiding superposition as much as possible. In general this situation arises when:

1. In spite of this high contrast fluid dosage the cecum has not been reached within approximately half an hour. Then transit is slow and the loops of the small intestine are always dilated. At first the roentgenogram does not show whether there is a mechanical obstruction or the dilatation is caused primarily by neurogenic or pharmacological factors. In a number of cases, it will appear during the examination that an organic stenosis is responsible for the slow passage.

2. The distal ileum is not clean due to food remnants or reflux of the colon contents. We have learned that reflux of colon contents often occurs in patients with colitis; apparently Bauhin's valve is then insufficient. The distal ileum is not thoroughly clean when the patient has not fasted, laxation is incomplete or sedatives or medication causing atonia have been given. In the latter case furthermore, transit is very slow, the lumen of the intestinal loops is widened and there is often superposition. Mixture of the colon contents with the contrast fluid in the distal ileum not only interferes with evaluation of the mucosal patterns in this area but often also seriously restricts the rate of transit. The extra water infusion causes the rate of transit to incrase and cleanses the distal ileum with the contrast fluid in front of the water. Only then can anatomical evalutation of the distal ileum be carried out. Fig. 40 shows that the mucosal patterns before and after the cleansing of the distal ileum can differ greatly so that the rash diagnosis 'reflux ileitis' must not be made too quickly.

3. By means of rapid administration of large amounts of contrast medium dilatation can be induced on the proximal side of stenoses which appear clinically as a light or intermittent subileus (pat. 30). The line of thought involved here can best be compared with that for hydration pyelography in pelvi-ureteric junction obstructions.

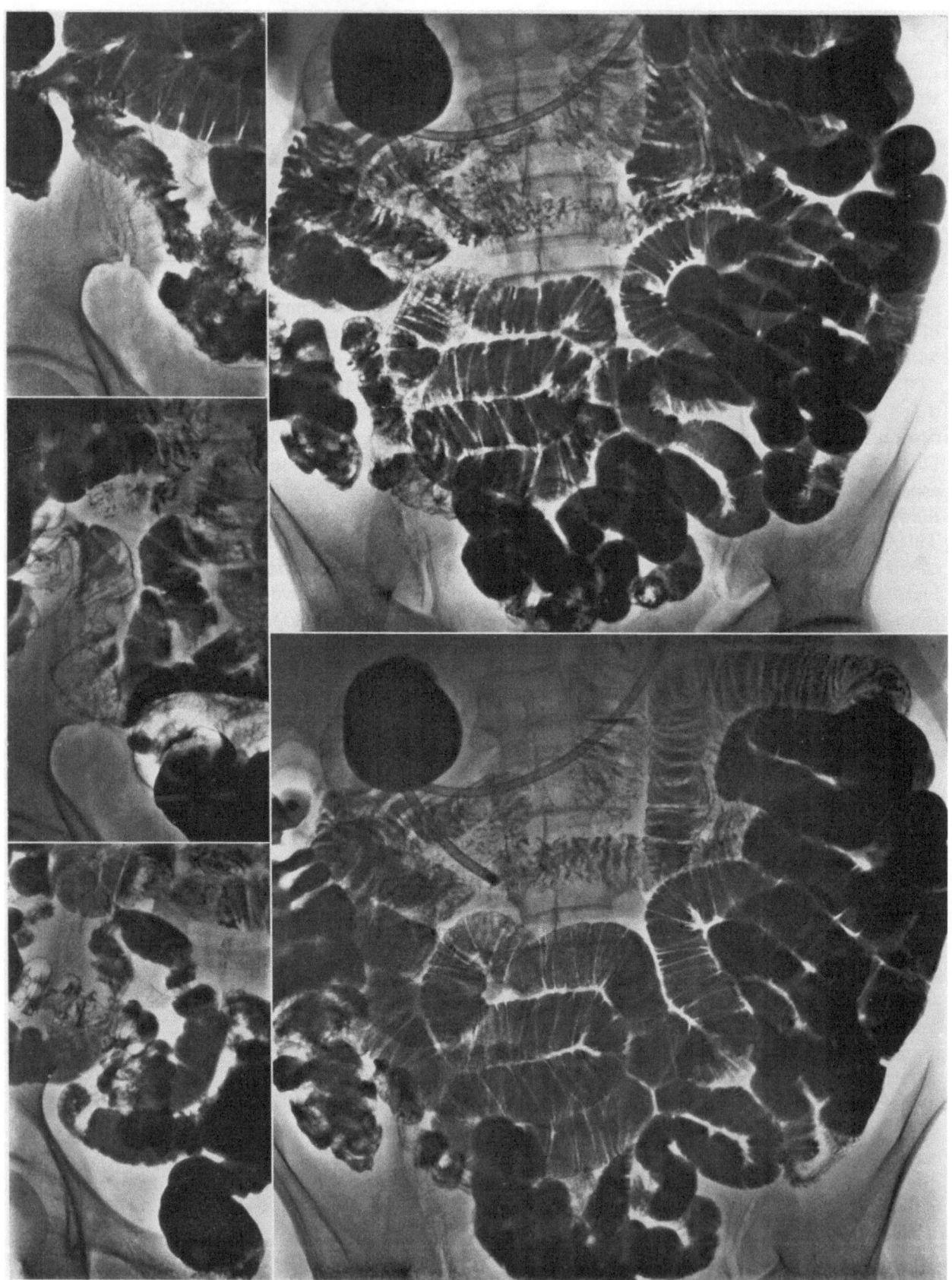

Fig. 29
A: 900 ml Microbar AZL (s.g. 1.32) + 600 ml water.
   An adhesive layer cannot be seen on the intestinal mucosa. The water has washed away the contrast fluid completely.

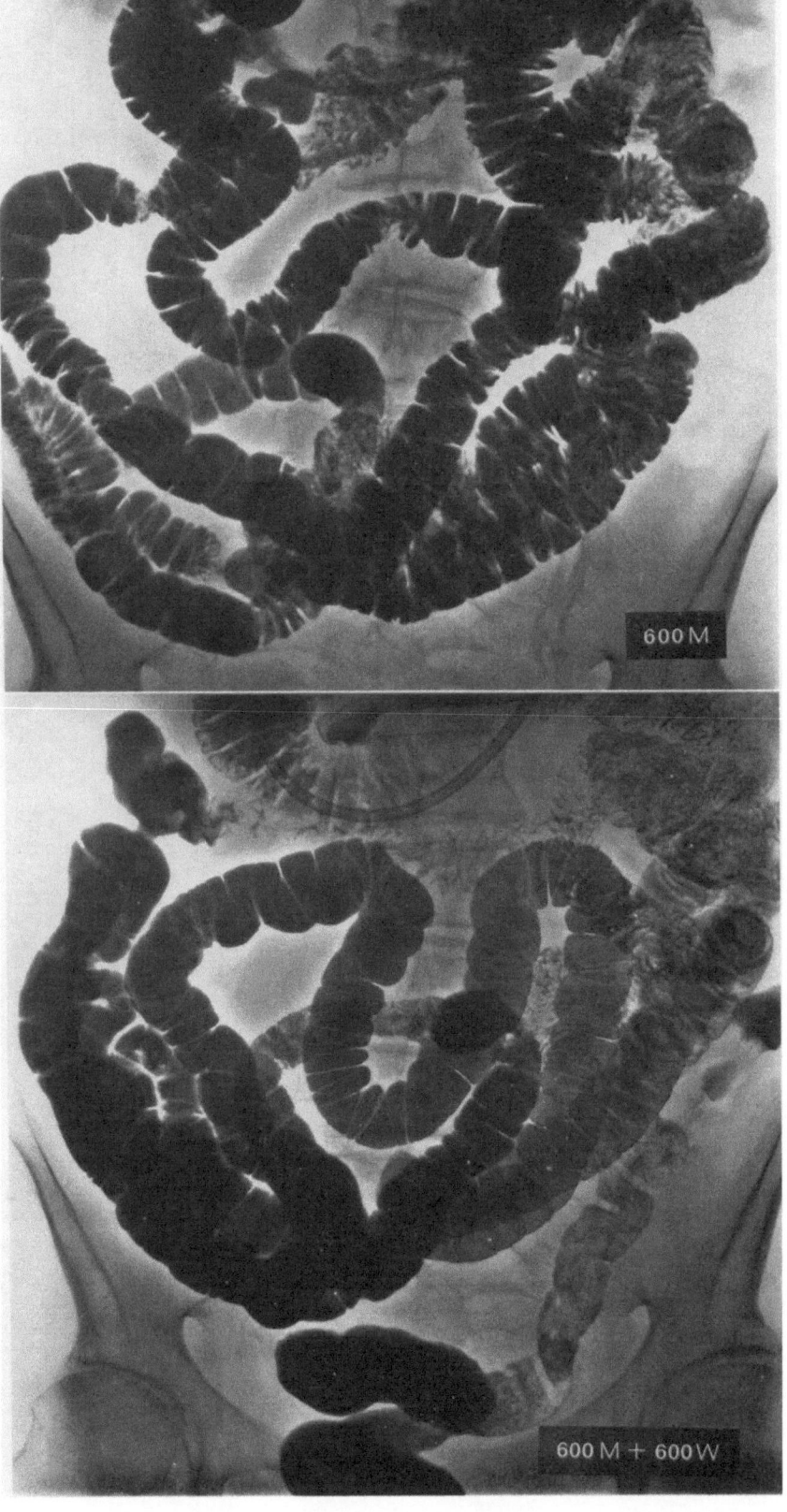

Fig. 29
B: 600 ml Micropaque (s.g. 1.26)
   + 600 ml water. A very thin
   layer of barium sulfate is left
   on the mucosa of the small
   intestine.

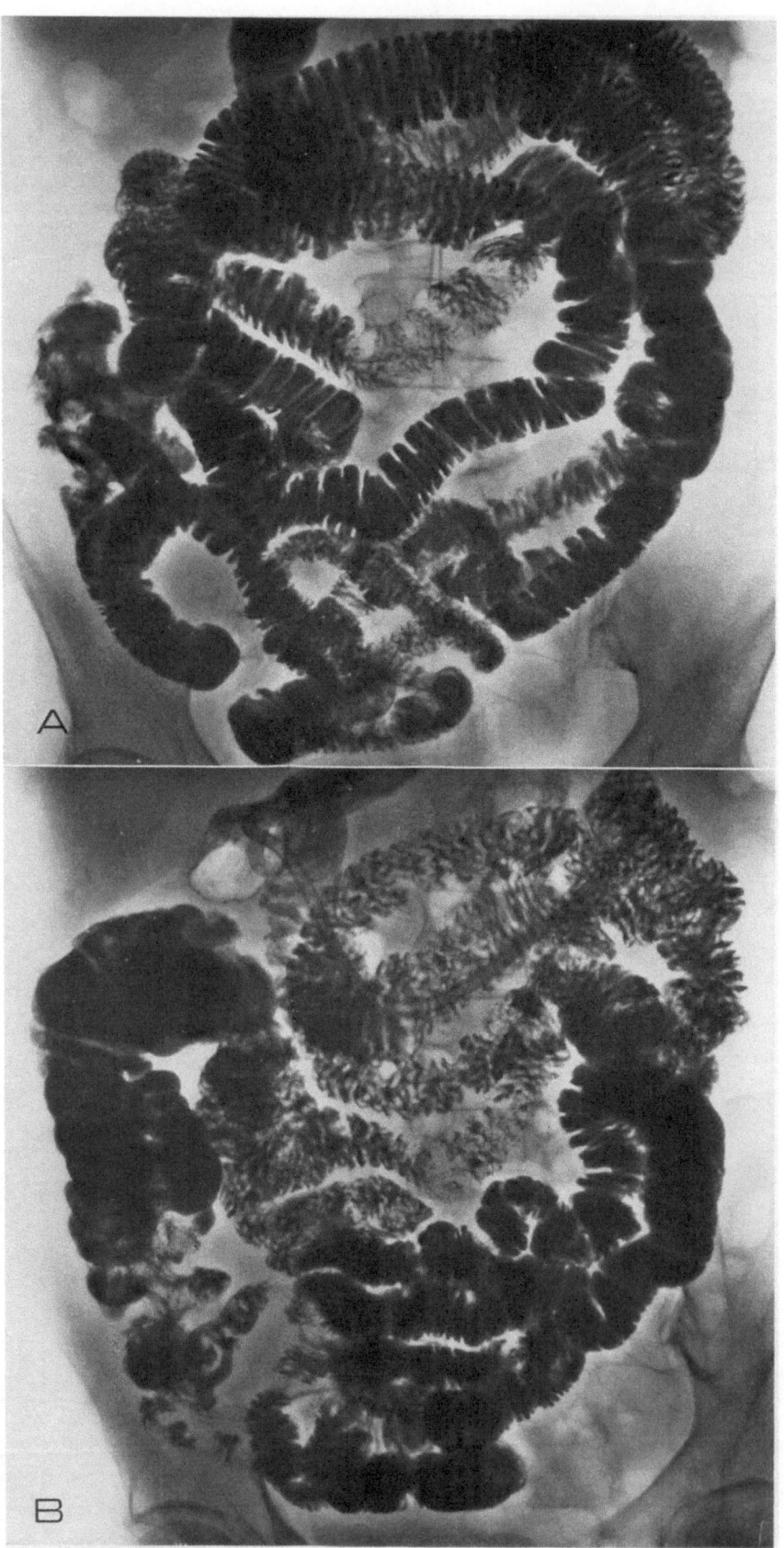

Fig. 30
600 ml Micropaque (s.g. 1.38)
+ 600 ml water.
A: at the end of the contrast
   medium infusion.
B: several minutes later.

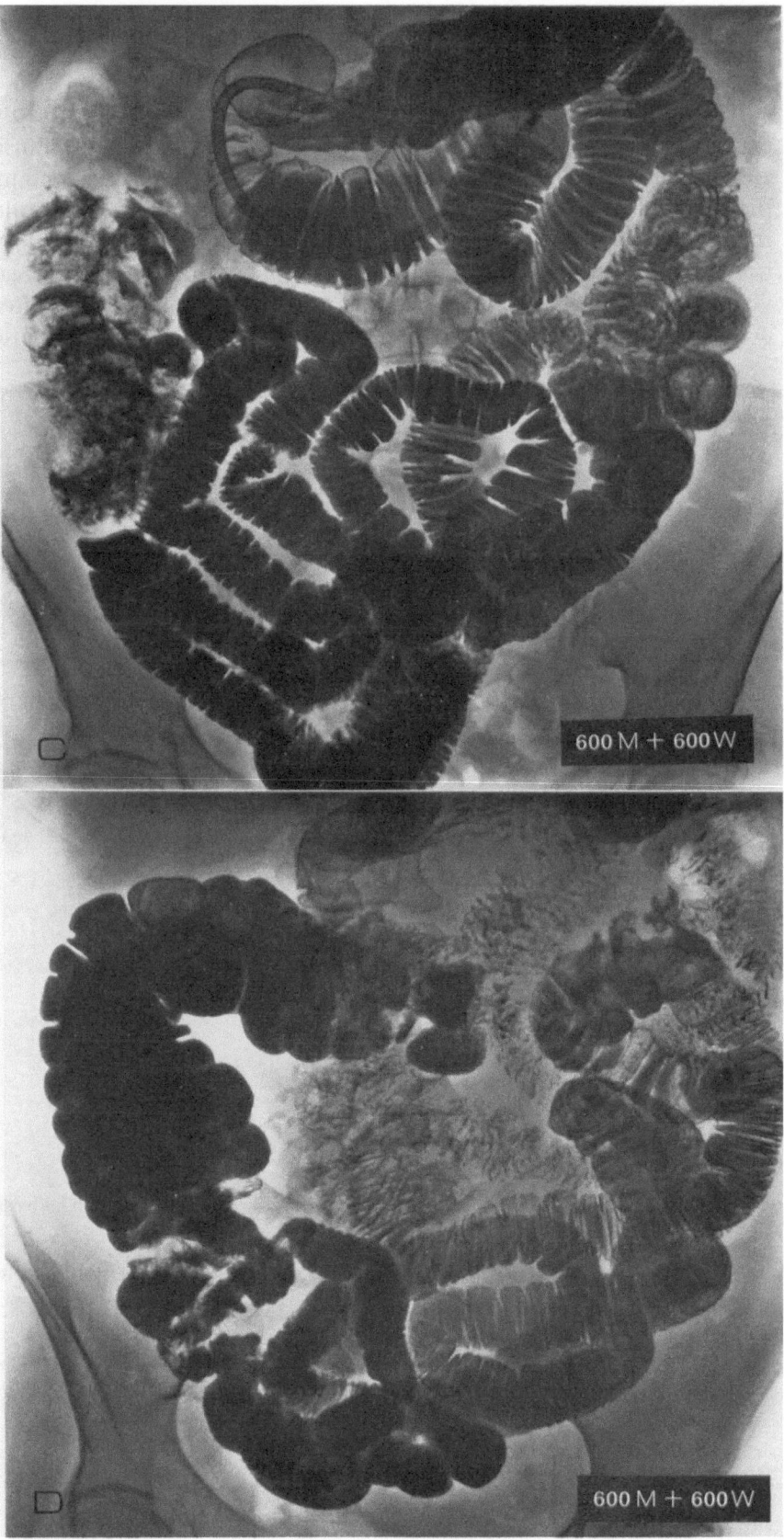

Fig. 30
c: at the end of the water
   infusion.
d: several minutes later. Contrast
   fluid has started to
   disintegrate in the jejunum.

For colitis patients whose complaints after a colectomy are due to a functional or anatomical narrowing of the anastomotic area, this stenosis can soon be diagnosed radiologically (13) (pat. 3 and pat. 10).

If there is no obstruction or dilatation, double-contrast exposures with air or water lengthen the examination by about 10 minutes. If there is an obstruction, the transit time can increase so that the entire examination lasts an hour, sometimes even longer. Large amounts of contrast medium shorten the length of the examination considerably. Until now we have as a rule not dared to administer more than 1800 ml; only two patients received 1200 ml contrast fluid plus 1200 ml water. Owing to the rapid transit, the contrast medium does not dehydrate in the ileum and it reaches the colon with a very low viscosity. We have found that large quantities of contrast fluid are already expelled 1 or 2 hours after administration and that even a large dosage does not cause constipation (fig. 31A).

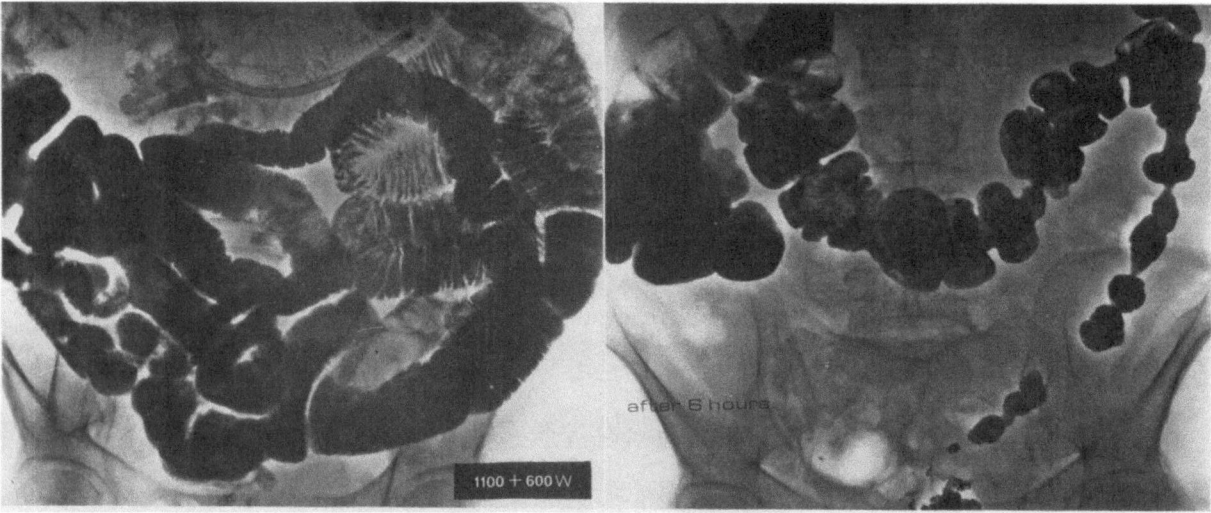

Fig. 31
A: barium residual in colon 6 hours after administration through tube of 1100 ml barium sulfate suspension (s.g. 1.32) and 600 ml water.

After the water infusion an increasing flocculation occurs in the zone between the water and the contrast column (fig. 31B). It is therefore sensible to regard the examination as ended soon after insufflation of air or water.

In the following chapter our experiences with this method of examination will be discussed. A number of photographs will be used to give an impression of the x-rays of the small intestine which can be obtained in this way.

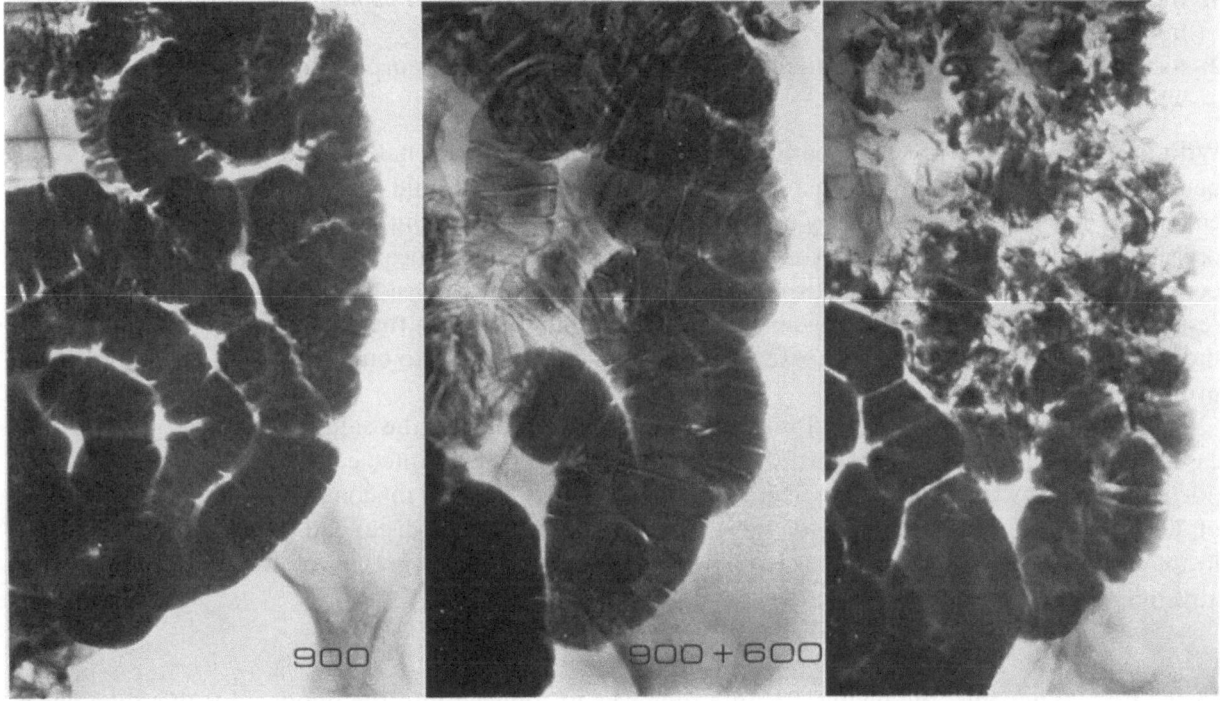

Fig. 31
B: disintegration of contrast fluid by mixing with an excess of water (flocculation).

IX
DISCUSSION OF PATIENTS

1. General considerations

The patients described in the following section can in no way be considered typical of the average radiological practice because:

1. there is a basic difference between the patients of a university hospital and those of a regional hospital.
2. to test our method of examination, the first 100 patients were purposefully selected, for reasons which will follow.

With a conventional x-ray examination of the small intestine, reasonably good mucosal patterns can be obtained in a large number of patients when a stable contrast fluid is used and gastric emptying is enhanced. The latter is achieved by administering a large dose of contrast medium, drugs to enhance peristalsis and placing the patient in the right lateral position. Since equally good or only slightly better results obtained with another technique would not be considered a true contribution, we restricted ourselves in so far as possible to those patients for whom the conventional examination of the small intestine did not produce satisfactory results or, according to our experience, would probably produce disappointing results.

The examination after duodenal intubation was carried out by the same radiologist or, in a few cases, under his supervision for the 100 patients described to guarantee consistency for the most important factors. All patients lay on their right side; they received 600 ml contrast fluid at a temperature of 20–24° C with a specific gravity of 1.25–1.3 through a tube. The distal end of the tube was located in the last 10 cm of the duodenum. Later we found that a specific gravity of 1.2–1.25 offers certain advantages (see chapter V.6).

I

In the first 20 patients, the pliable Rehfuss tube was introduced into the duodenum; this tube has a metal, olive-shaped end with several holes or grooves. Initially it cost an hour, and sometimes even longer; however once curling of the tube in the stomach was restricted by passing a feed line from a Seldinger catheter through the tube, this time was reduced to half an hour. The patients lay on their right side and were not given any drugs to enhance peristalsis. Now and then, progress was checked under the fluoroscope.

For one of the 20 patients, intubation was not possible so that the infusion examination had to be abandoned. The remaining 19 patients received the contrast fluid in an average of 11.5 minutes (extreme values 3 and 20 minutes).

Reflux into the stomach was seen in only one patient of this group. In this case, an attempt was made to stimulate gastric emptying by an intravenous injection of 10 mg Primperan, without success.

In spite of the long time needed for intubation, on the average more than 30 minutes, and the use of not more than 600 ml contrast fluid, the average total length of the examination for these 19 patients was still only 71 minutes. Seven patients from this first group had had a conventional gastro-intestinal transit examination 10 days to 2 years previously, which lasted an average of 5 hours and 40 minutes.

II

Our experience with the first 20 patients led us to suspect that the time required for intubation into the duodenum could be shortened if the feed line through the tube were more rigid than for the Seldinger catheter. Purchase of the Bilbao-Dotter unit therefore resulted in a definite improvement in the intubation technique, mainly due to the more rigid feed line. The results obtained with this unit in 81 patients were very favourable. With the help of the x-ray technician, the patient first swallowed 75 cm of the tube; the time required by the radiologist to position the tube correctly was then 13–15 min. for 5 patients, 9–12 min. for 7 patients, 6–8 min. for 4 patients and 3–5 min. for the rest.

Intubation was successful in all patients of this group, although the more pliable Rehfuss tube had to be used in 4 patients with a steerhornstomach since the Bilbao-tube curled in the cardiac area even when the patient stood erect. In these cases, intubation of the pliable tube was successful when the patient lay on his right side and leaned slightly forward so that the heavy olive-shaped metal end of the Rehfuss tube fell down toward the pyloric canal.

The 81 patients received 600 ml contrast medium administered in 3–5 minutes. Supplementary administration of contrast fluid or water took place at the same rate. For these 81 patients, the average examination lasted only 36 minutes, including the time necessary for duodenal intubation and double-contrast exposures.

For 46 patients, one single administration of 600 ml contrast medium was sufficient; for 15 of these patients the examination also included double-contrast exposures with air.

Thirty-five patients received a second dose of contrast medium averaging 500 ml (extreme values 300 and 600 ml).

For 21 patients, the examination also included a water infusion: 2 patients received 1200 ml, two 300 ml, four 400 ml and the rest 600 ml. Of the 21 patients given a water infusion, 7 had already received a second dosage of contrast medium.

It was striking that in 11 of the 81 patients, reflux of the contrast fluid into the stomach was observed while it occurred only once in the first group of 19 patients. Probably this can be explained by the difference in the rate of administration: in group II it was administered much faster than in group I. Within 5 minutes eight of these 11 patients received a second dose of 600 ml contrast medium containing 20 ml Primperan. Two patients received a second dose of only 300 ml because the cecum had almost been reached; the colon had already been reached in 1 patient and therefore a supplementary dosage was not necessary.

The average total examination time for these 11 patients was exactly 1 hour and thus obviously lengthened. It was also remarkable that due to the increased rate of flow of more than 600 ml contrast fluid, not one patient showed distinct signs of flocculation or segmentation, regardless of the contrast medium used (Microbar AZL, Bario-dif or Micropaque). The contrast medium chosen for this examination method is of only secondary importance. It is obvious that a stable contrast fluid will still provide good results even when the infusion rate is low. In addition, because of the better buffer action, a lower total dosage will suffice. Furthermore it is clear that the best double-contrast exposures are obtained when the contrast medium has the highest possible viscosity at a certain specific gravity so that an infusion rate of 100 ml per minute through our infusion system is still possible.

Thirty-three of the 81 patients had previously been examined by the conventional method; for 19 patients the examination of the small intestine had taken place less than a year ago and the average transit time was 3.5 hours. For the other 14 patients, the previous examination was more than a year ago and the average transit was 5.25 hours (Sorbitol was not yet used at that time).

Two methods of examination can best be compared when each patient is examined by both techniques within a short period of time. In view of the radiation involved, we did not use this principle

However the fortunate situation did arise that for 11 patients a repeat examination using the infusion technique was indicated.

For these 11 patients, an average of 12 days before the infusion a conventional transit examination had been carried out using 300 ml contrast fluid and 30 ml Sorbitol. The last films were taken an average of 4 hours after the patient had received the contrast medium (extreme values 1 and 8 hours). In 2 cases, the colon had not yet been reached although the examination lasted an entire day. During the conventional examination, seven of these 11 patients showed such heavy thickening and segmentation of the contrast fluid in the ileum that anatomical evaluation was impossible (figs. 34, 75, 74c, d).

For the remaining 4 patients, the average transit time for the conventional examination was only 105 minutes. In the distal ileum, the contrast fluid had then more or less retained its homogeneous structure and low viscosity so that reasonably clear mucosal patterns were seen (figs. 45, 52a).

It is obvious that observation of anatomical abnormalities of the mucous membrane of the small intestine depends mainly upon the characteristics of the contrast medium at the moment the roentgenograms are made.

2. Patients

I

Eighteen patients had Crohn's disease (histological verification from surgical specimens or rectal biopsy); in 11 of these cases the distal ileum, cecum and a part of the ascending colon had already been resected. The remaining 7 patients had Crohn's disease of the colon; in 5 patients, the colon had been removed. Three of these 5 patients had an ileo-rectal anastomosis, 2 an ileostomy.

Radiological examination showed a recurrence or stenosis in 8 of the 16 patients treated by surgery. Three of these 8 patients had had a conventional examination of the small intestine less than one year ago; they will be discussed first.

Patient 1: Status after ileo-cecal resection. The examination after duodenal intubation shows a recurrence in the last loop of the ileum. During a conventional examination eight months ago the last loop appeared to be completely normal. Fig. 32 reveals that the mucosal pattern of the ileum is more detailed by the infusion technique than the conventional transit examination. During the latter examination, the contrast medium probably acquired a higher viscosity due to fluid absorption and therefore could not penetrate the small folds.

Patient 2: Status after total colectomy: The infusion lasted 10 minutes and revealed a 2 cm stenosis in the area of the A.P. (verified surgically). There is a moderate prestenotic dilatation of the ileum; the mucosal folds are coarse. Four weeks previously a conventional examination was carried out which lasted 70 minutes. Although in this examination a stenosis in the area of the A.P. with a prestenotic dilatation of the ileum was also seen, it was not interpreted as such.

Patient 3: The findings were especially interesting for a very thin 52-year-old patient who had had a total colectomy because of a suspected ulcerative colitis. Although 600 ml contrast medium was administered twice by infusion, the ileo-rectal anastomosis had not yet been reached after 1 hour. It was however noticed that the ileum loops increased in width in the distal direction and that they contained so much feces that pictures of the anastomosis suitable for anatomical evaluation could not be obtained; this led to the diagnosis of a stenosis (figs. 33a-d). The conventional examination one year earlier lasted 8 hours and showed 'mucosal patterns' in the lower right abdomen which were interpreted as definite pathological ileal loops and fistulous tracts (fig. 34a). Now however there was

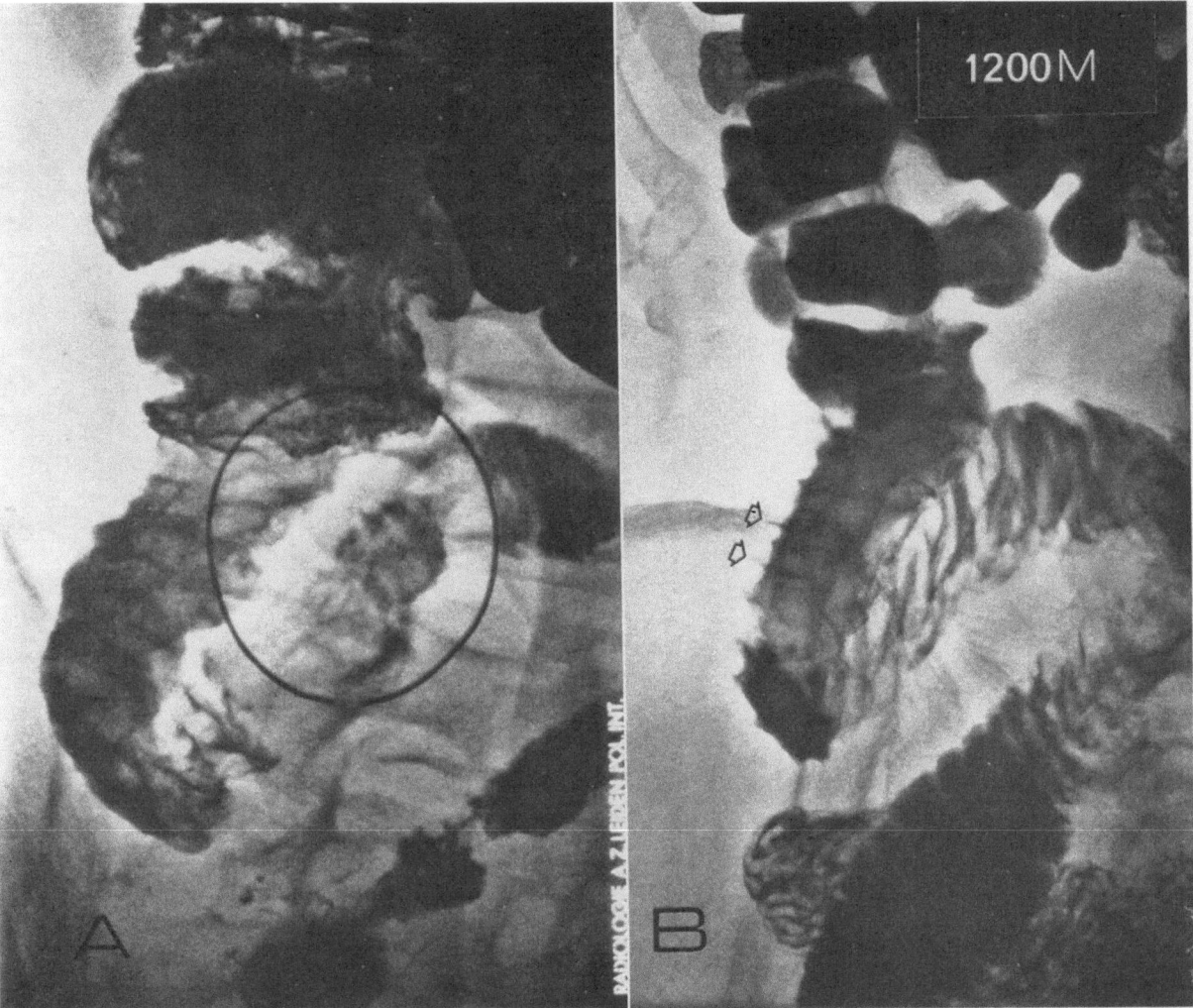

Fig. 32
Pat. 1: Crohn's disease.
A: conv.; splotchy picture of contrast column. Last ileum loop before anastomosis with ascending colon shows smooth outline. Few mucosal folds visible.
B: inf; homogeneous structure of contrast column. The narrow spaces between the clearly visible mucosal folds are filled with contrast fluid.

absolutely no supporting evidence; in particular the configurations of the intestinal loops in the right lower abdomen were completely different and reasonably normal (fig. 33B).

Although highly improbable and contrary to the clinical course, it was presumed that the pathological intestinal loops and fistulous tracts seen previously had now disappeared. Therefore it was decided to repeat the examination using the conventional technique. It is quite surprising that 6 hours after administration of the contrast medium, this examination appeared to reveal practically the same 'pathology', due to the segmentation of the contrast fluid, as the examination of one year ago. Furthermore a highly exposed film of one single loop showed that the contrast fluid was no longer as homo-

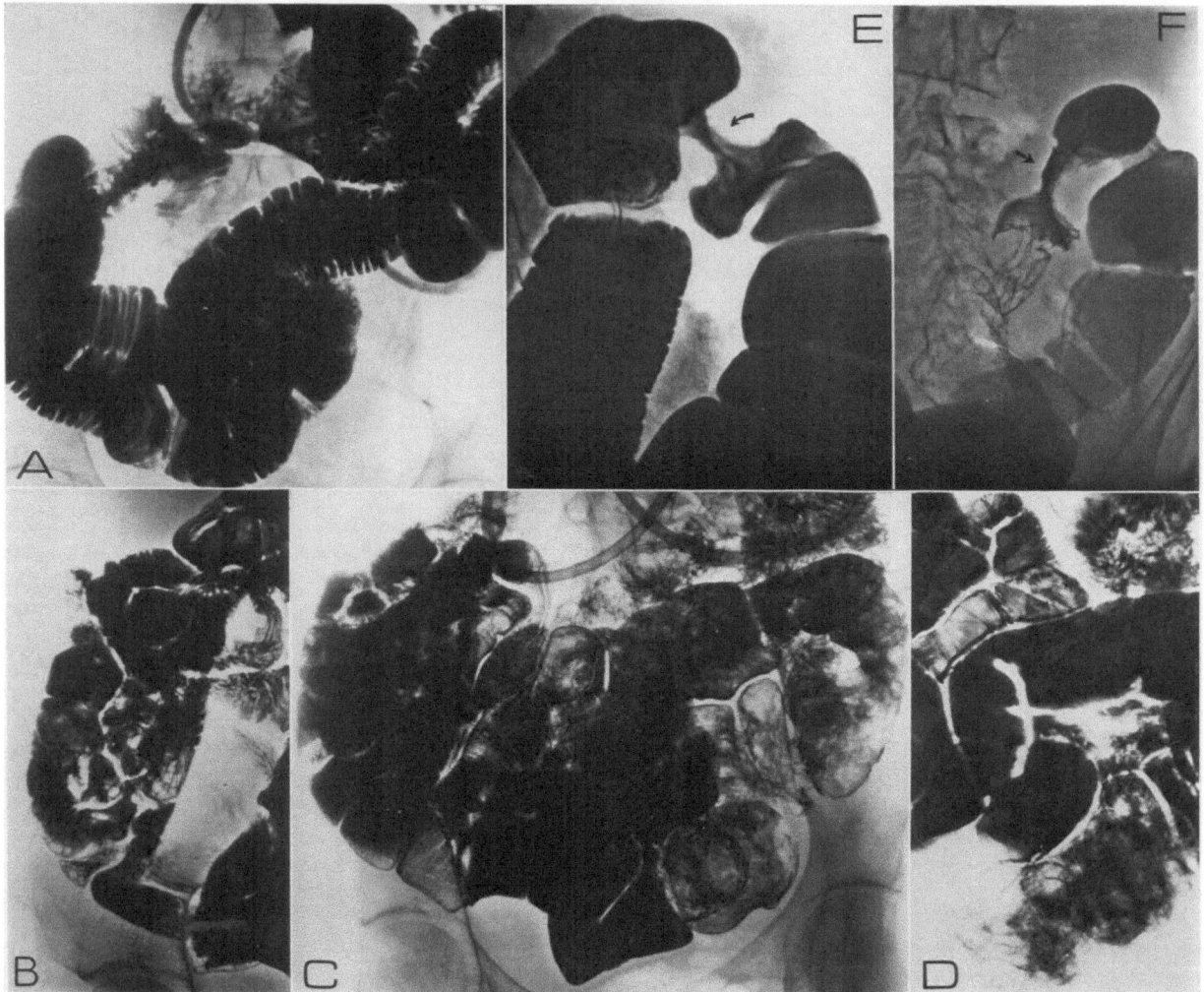

Fig. 33
Pat. 3: Ileo-rectal anastomosis, Crohn's disease
A, B, C, D: inf; 1200 ml Microbar AZL (s.g. 1.32). Examination time 1 hour. Slow passage, wide loops, extensive fecal contamination.
E, F: rectal filling with contrast fluid. Narrow anastomosis and marked increase in width of ileum.

geneous as the weaker exposure suggested (fig. 34B). Since rectoscopy to 40 cm revealed no stenosis, the patient was treated conservatively for some time. Surgery took place only after rectal administration of contrast fluid on two separate occasions revealed the stenosis without reservation (figs. 33E, F).

Pathological anatomical examination of the resected section demonstrated Crohn's disease instead of ulcerative colitis.

In two other patients, the radiological examination using the infusion technique showed a stenotic recurrence; however since the conventional examination took place more than a year ago, comparison of the results is not considered feasible. In *patient 4*, the 4 hour transit examination 1.5 years ago resulted in heavy segmentation of the contrast fluid (figs. 35C, D), as did the 2 hour examination of

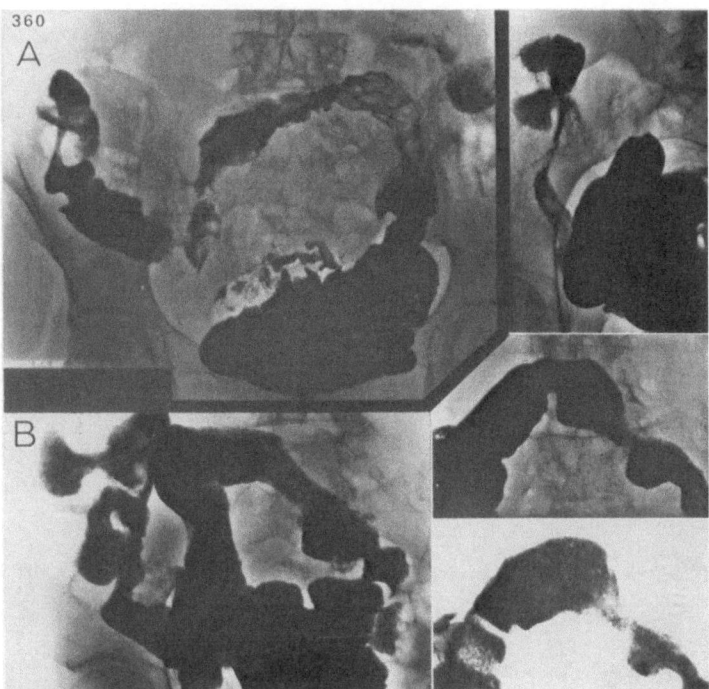

Fig. 34
Pat. 3:
A: conventional transit examination 1 year ago lasted 8 hours. diagnosis: path. ileum loops and fistulous tracts.
B: conv. examination repeated recently (300 ml orally). Pictures (unrealistic) identical to 1 year ago.

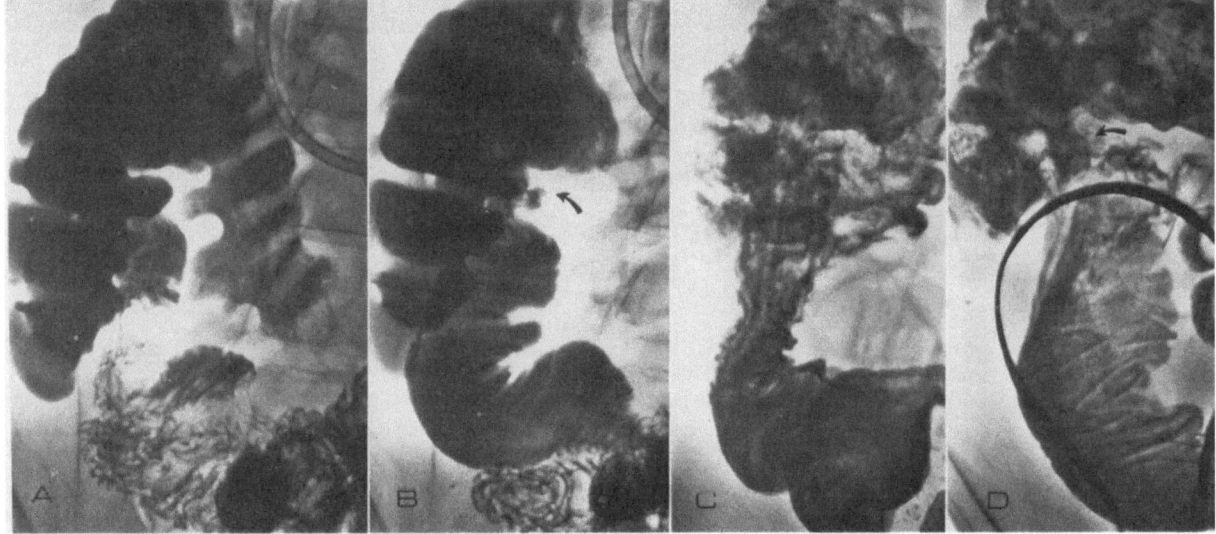

Fig. 35
Pat. 4: Ileo-transversostomy, Crohn's disease.
A, B: inf; stenosis of the anastomosis.
C, D: conv; width of ileum also increased. Disintegration of contrast fluid.

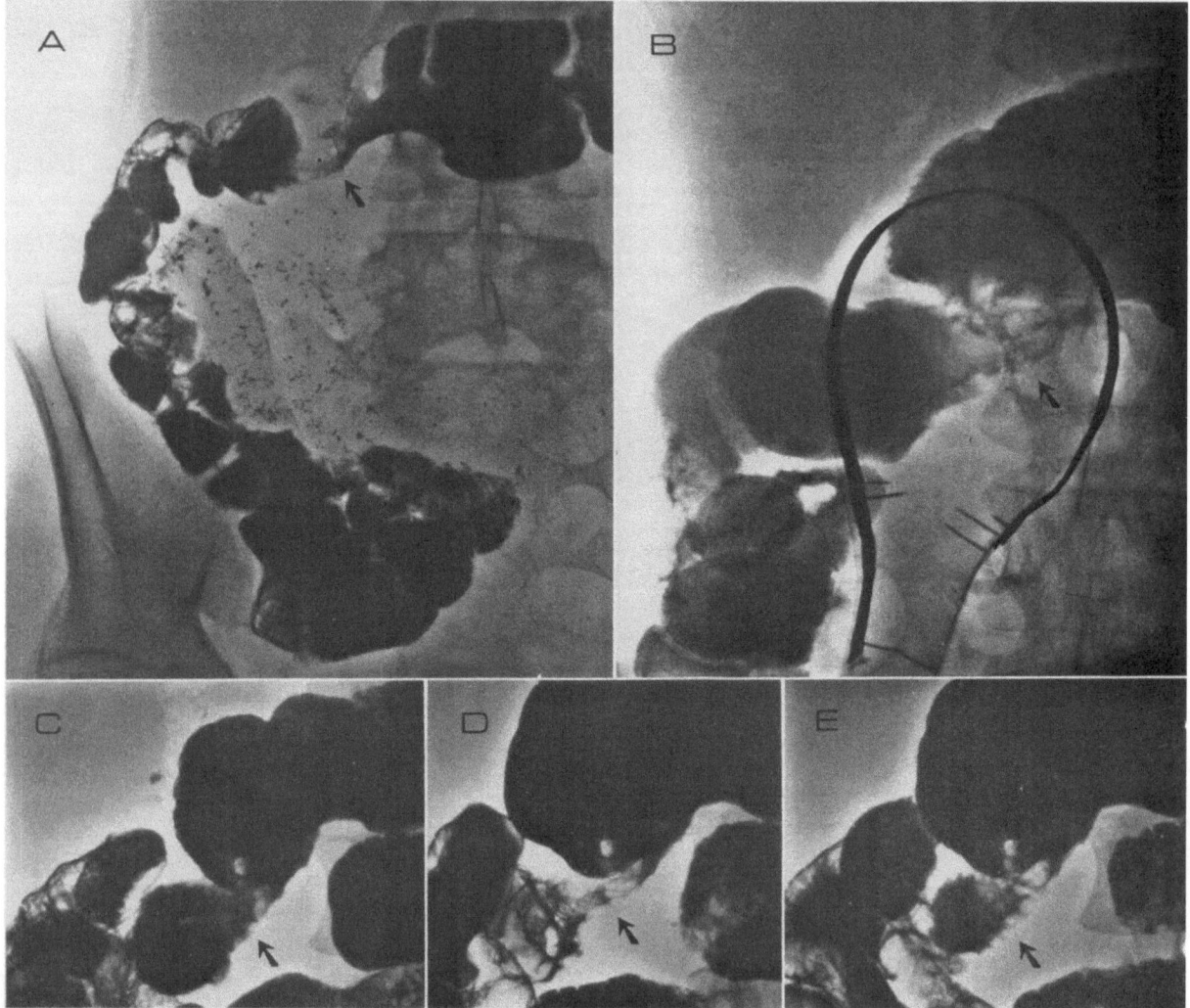

Fig. 36
Pat. 5: Ileo-transversostomy, Crohn's disease.
A: conv; pronounced disintegration of contrast fluid.
B: rectal contrast filling. Narrow anastomosis.
C, D, E: inf; stenotic recurrence of Crohn's disease in region of anastomosis.

patient 5 two years ago (fig. 36A). Neither of these examinations revealed abnormalities, although a subsequent colon examination of patient 5 did (fig. 36 B).

For the remaining 3 patients showing a recurrence, a previous examination was not available for comparison. Two of these 3 patients are however worth mentioning.

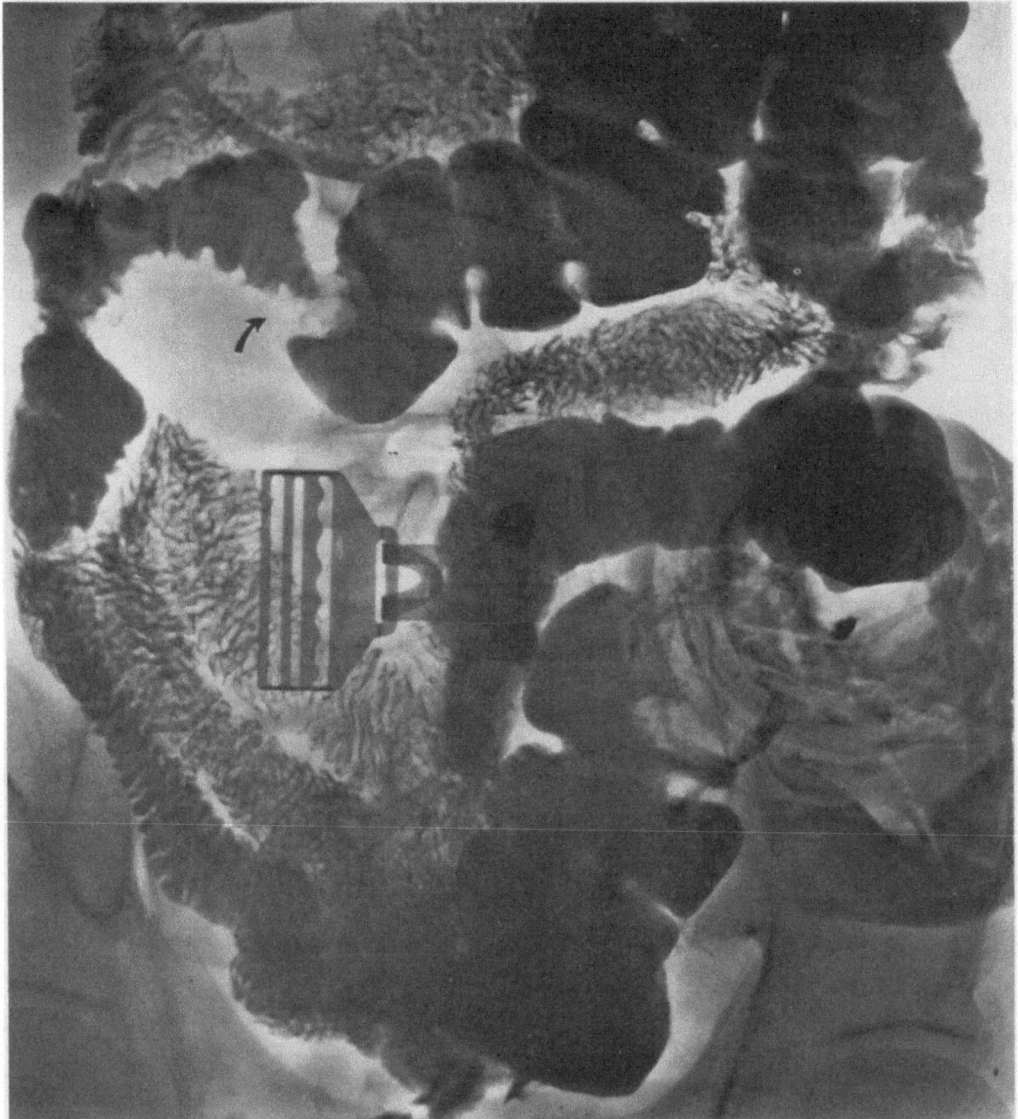

Fig. 37
Pat. 6: Status after ileo-transversostomy, Crohn's disease. Stenotic recurrence in region of anastomosis. There is little left of the ileum. The anastomosis was reached 1 minute after the contrast medium infusion was started. 600 ml Microbar AZL (s.g. 1.32).

Patient 6: Status after ileo-cecal resection, recurrence in the last section of the ileum. In this patient, it was striking that the anastomosis between the ileum and the transverse colon, was reached one minute after the contrast infusion was started. A study of the x-rays clearly indicates that the remaining small intestine consists almost entirely of jejunal loops and that there is practically no ileum left (fig. 37).

Patient 7: Status after ileo-cecal resection, recurrence in the last section of the ileum (figs. 38A, B). Because the examination was so short (15 minutes from duodenum to anus), the viscosity of the contrast fluid was very low when the rectum was reached and there was no sign of flocculation. It is certainly due to these 2 factors that an excellent barium filling of the pararectal fistulous tracts was seen at the end of the transit examination (figs. 38C-F). Communication of these fistulous tracts with the rectum was therefore assumed without reservation, although it was less clearly visible than on the subsequent fistulogram (fig. 38G).

Two of the 18 patients were not operated on; they both had Crohn's disease of the colon which for a long time was believed to be an ulcerative colitis.

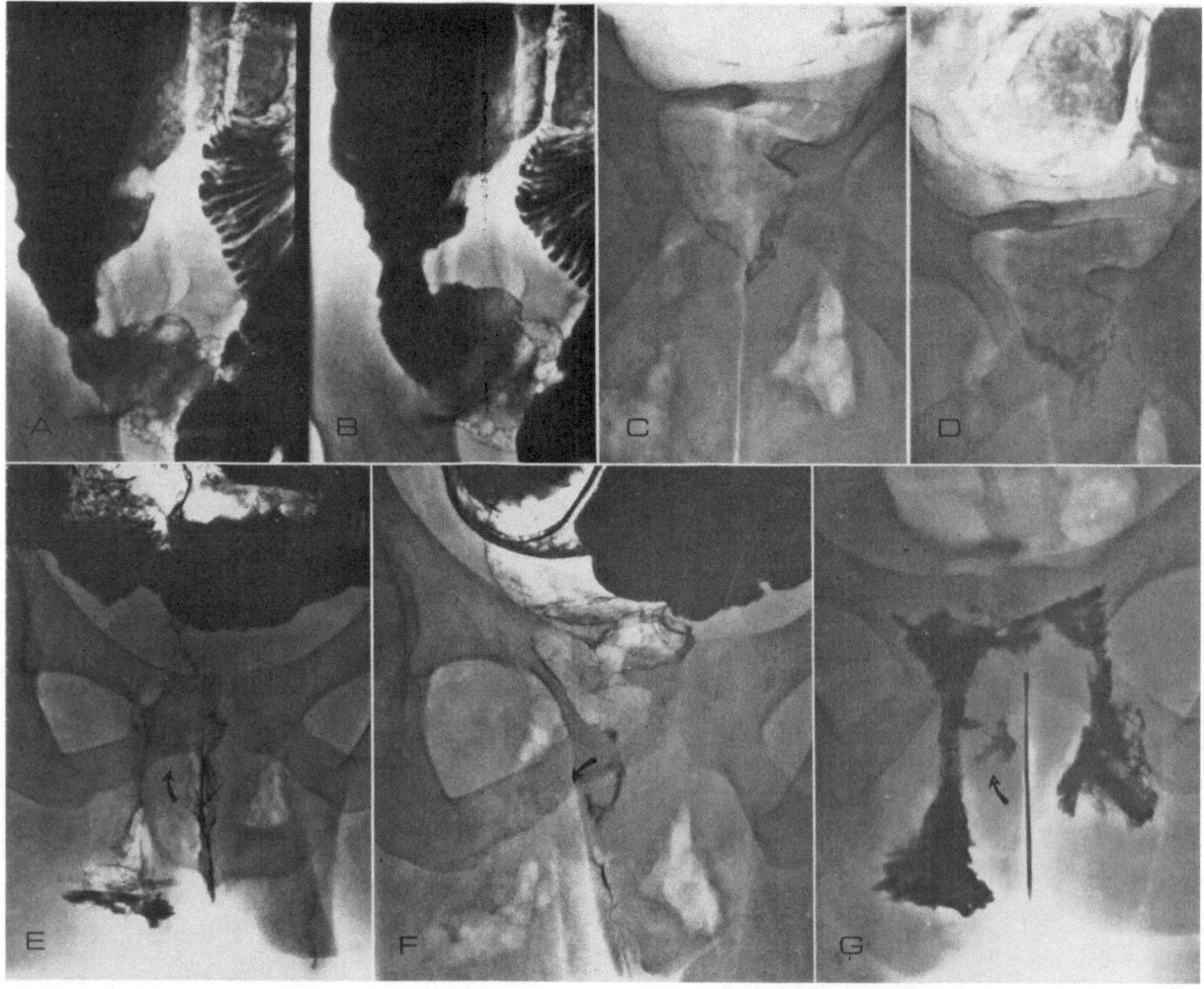

Fig. 38
Pat. 7: status after ileo-cecal resection, Crohn's disease.
A, B: Stenotic recurrence in distal ileum.
C, D, E, F: After oral air insufflation, clear pictures of para-rectal fistulous tracts are obtained.
G: Fistulogram.

Patient 8: was a 14-year-old girl. The radiological examination after duodenal intubation revealed local mucosal abnormalities in the distal ileum; the 'cobble-stone' appearance suggests Crohn's disease (fig. 39A). The conventional examination 5 months earlier had lasted 7 hours in spite of the use of transit accelerating drugs; no abnormalities were found (fig. 39B).

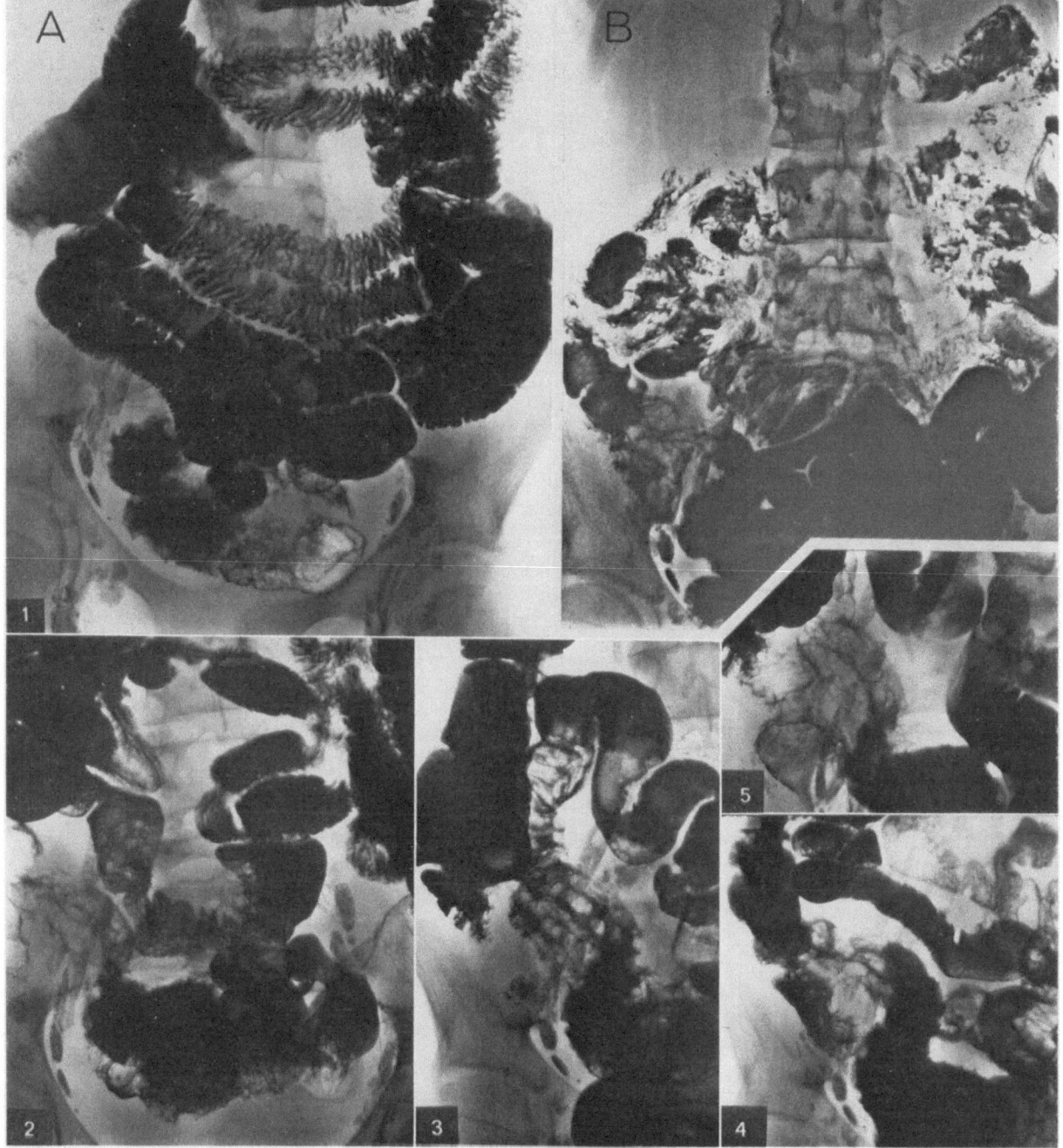

Fig. 39
Pat. 8: M. Crohn.
A: inf; 400 ml Micropaque (s.g. 1.38), 'cobble stone' pattern in last ileal loop.
B: conv; 5 months earlier. Disintegration of contrast fluid. No abnormalities were found.

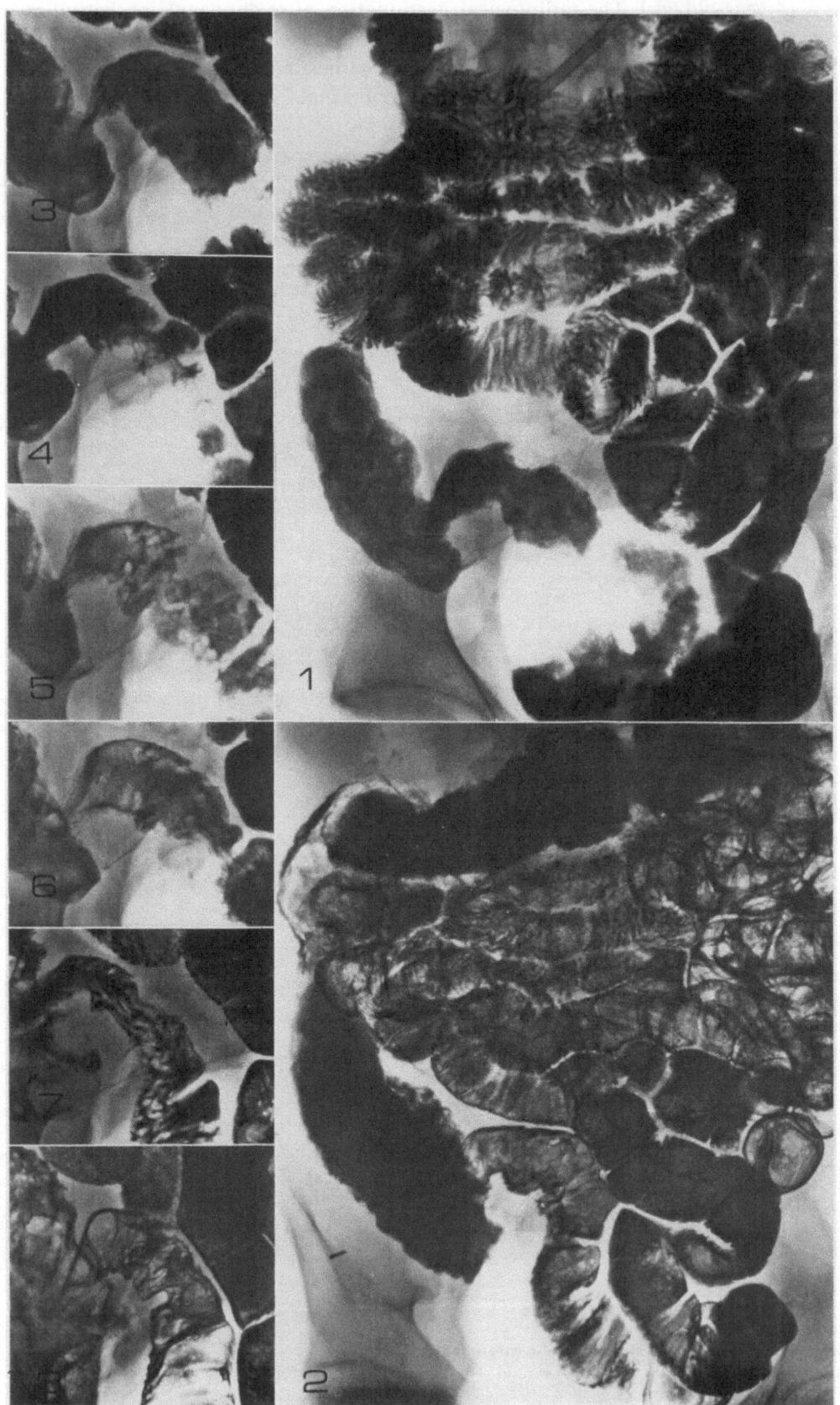

Fig. 40

Patient 9 was a 20-year-old young man. The radiological examination after duodenal intubation initially showed an absence of mucosal folds in the distal ileum and a highly irregular structure of the contrast fluid. In the course of the examination it appeared however that this structure was caused by reflux of the colon contents. Finally normal mucosal patterns were seen with no convincing abnormalities, not even with double-contrast exposures (fig. 40). Quite sometime later, after the air had disappeared completely out of the small intestine, the contrast fluid showed clear signs of flocculation and segmentation, as did the examination 4 years ago (fig. 41).

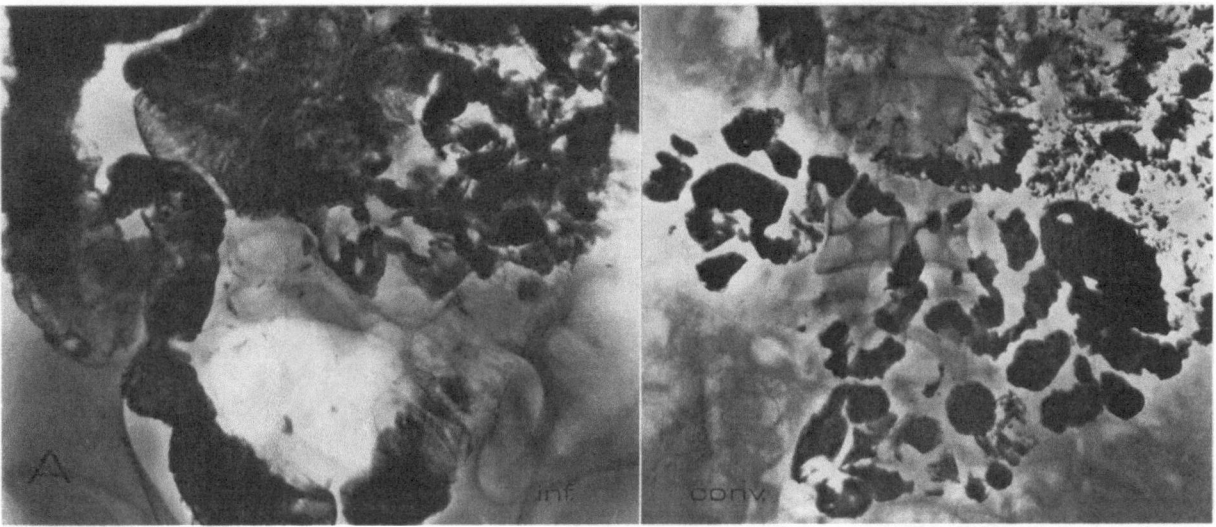

Fig. 41
Pat. 9: Disintegration of contrast fluid on conventional transit examination and at the end of the examination after duodenal intubation.

Fig. 40
Pat. 9: Crohn's disease of the colon.

Inf; 600 ml Micropaque (s.g. 1.38). Reflux of colon contents into ileum. Exposures 1 and 3 show *Pseudo-refluxileitis.* On later exposures and after air insufflation, abnormalities can no longer be seen.

II

Ten patients with colitis or sigmoiditis underwent a radiological examination of the small intestine. Two of these 10 patients had had a colectomy and both had an ile-orectal anastomosis. In one case the rectal stump was very short and a marked narrowing of the anastomosis had occurred with a pronounced prestenotic dilatation of the ileum (*patient 10*, fig. 42). For the other patient, as well as the remaining 8 patients, no abnormalities could be demonstrated.

It is striking that in 5 of the 10 patients of this group, the loops of the small intestine were slihgtly wider and the transit time was clearly lengthened. The two patients with the ileo-rectal anastomosis are included in these 5; in a third patient adhesions were found and in the other 2, reflux of the colon contents into the ileum was noted.

The average examination time for the 10 colitis patients was approximately 1 hour and therefore considerably lengthened; the average dose of contrast medium was 950 ml and therefore agreed fairly well with the total average of 900 ml for all 100 patients.

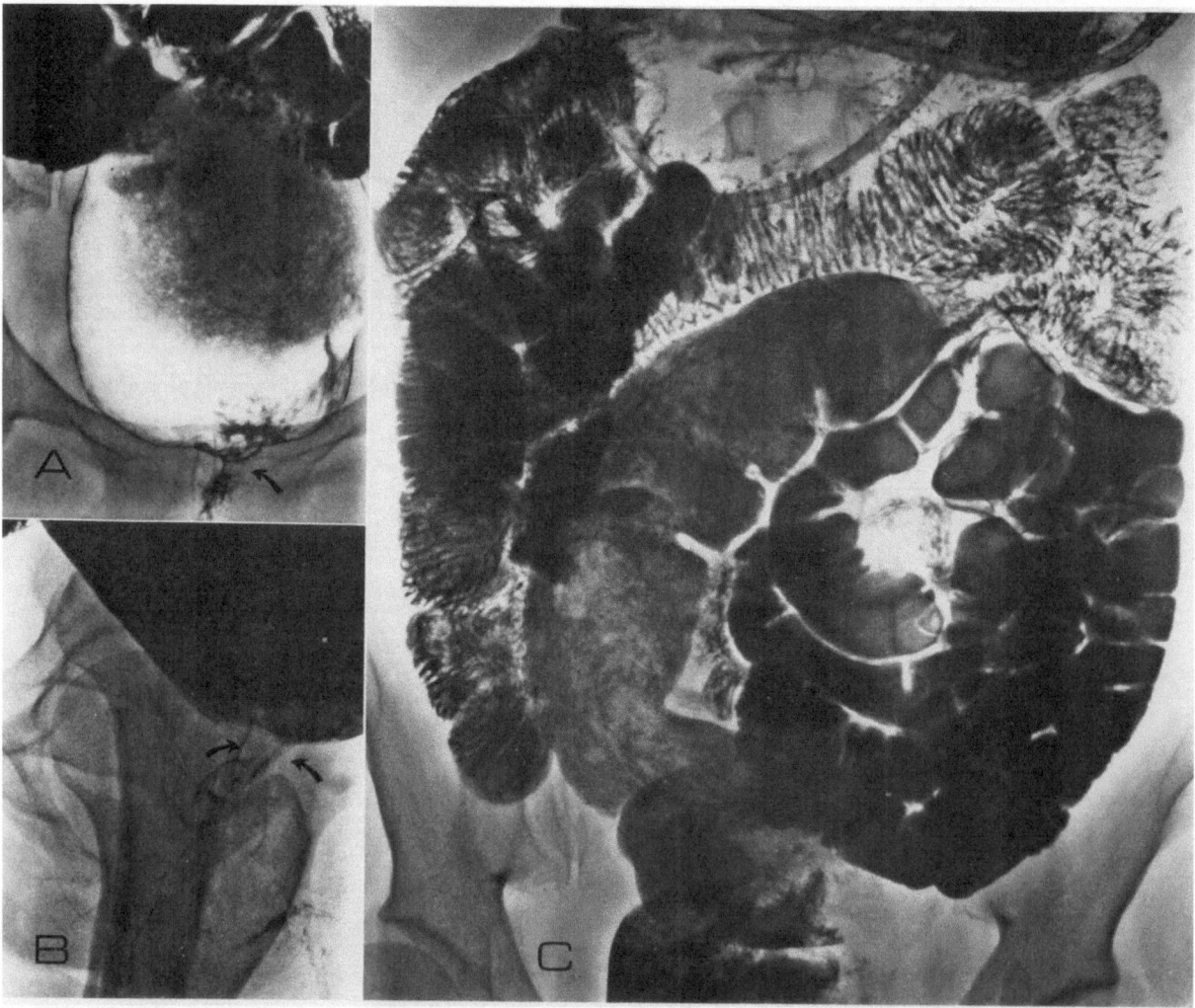

Fig. 42
Pat. 10: Ileo-rectal anastomosis, colitis (ulcerative?)
inf; 600 ml Microbar AZL (s.g. 1.32) + 400 ml water.
Pronounced stenosis in the region of the anus with prestenotic dilatation of ileum.
Surgical findings revealed anastomosis 8 cm before anus; the stenosis was 5 cm long.

Only 2 of the 10 patients had had conventional transit examinations earlier; for one this was 3 years ago, for the other 6 weeks. The present examination lasted a half hour and 2 hours for these two patients in contrast to 6.5 and 12 hours for the conventional method. Fig. 43 (*patient 11*) and fig. 44 (*patient 12*) show the differences in the results obtained for the distal ileum; abnormalities were not found.

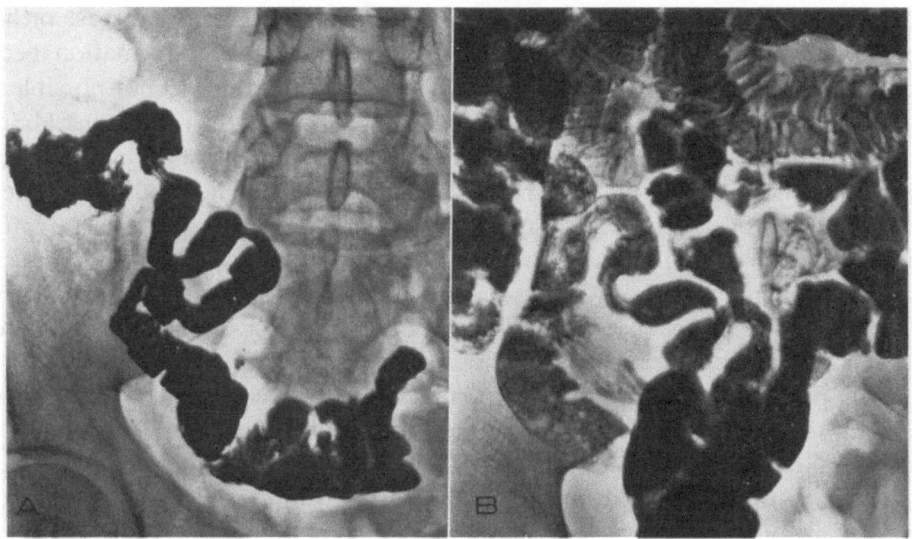

Fig. 43
Pat. 11: Colitis.
A: conv; 3 years previously, 6.5 hours.
B: inf; 600 cc. Microbar AZL (s.g. 1.32), 30 min.

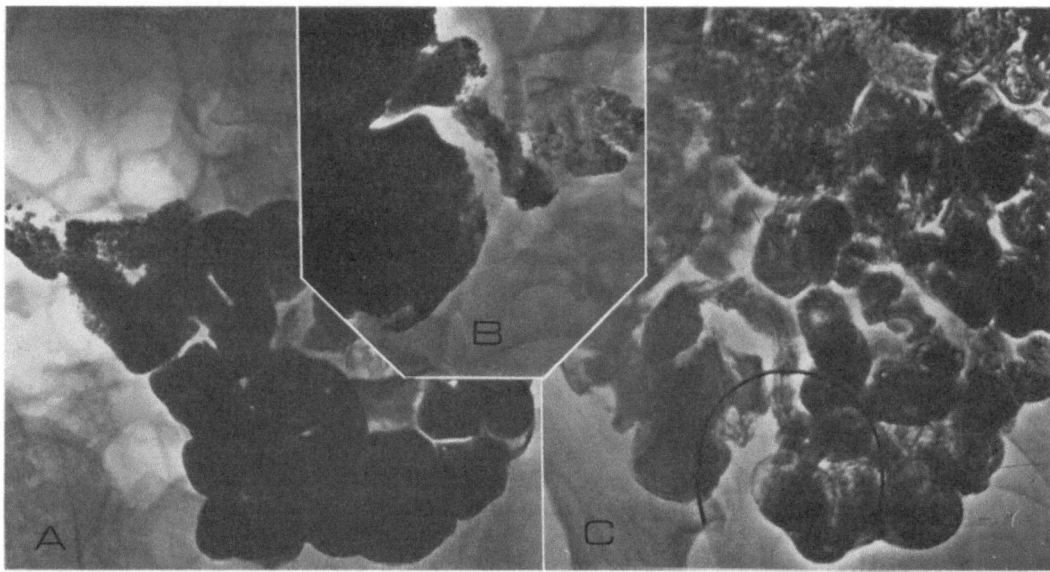

Fig. 44
Pat. 12: Colitis.
A, B: conv; 6 weeks previously, 300 ml Microbar AZL orally. Transit time 12 hours. Disintegration and thickening of contrast fluid.
C: inf; 600 ml Microbar AZL (s.g. 1.32). Administered in 15 min. Transit time 2 hours. Good mucosal patterns; filling of last ileum loop.

III

For another 10 patients, the examination of the small intestine was carried out because the presence of an intra-abdominal or para-rectal infiltration or fistulous process was known or presumed. Only two patients of this group had been examined previously by the conventional method.

In *patient 13*, a large fistulous process in the lower right abdomen was already diagnosed 2 weeks previously by means of a conventional examination and ascribed to Crohn's disease or herring worm disease. Although the infusion technique provided more anatomical information because of the larger and faster supply of contrast medium, a more specific diagnosis was not possible (fig. 45).

Patient 14 was a 20-year-old female who had complained of pain in the right lower abdomen for the past several years. Her brother had Crohn's disease. The patient had had a 6 hour conventional transit examination 2 years earlier and no abnormalities were found. The exposures made at that time showed heavy flocculation and segmentation of the contrast fluid (figs. 46A, B). The infusion examination lasted 20 minutes; 600 ml contrast medium was used followed by 400 ml water. On several exposures local irregular mucosal folds were seen in the ileum approximately 50 cm before the valve of Bauhin; the significance of this observation was not clear (figs. 46C-F). Two months later this ileum loop was re-examined and convincing abnormalities were no longer visible (fig. 46G). Apparently the previous observations were temporary mucosal abnormalities which probably would not have been seen if the infusion technique had not been used. The future will show whether this was actually an initial abnormality due to Crohn's disease in an even earlier stage than in patient 33. Since the x-rays of the second examination showed absolutely no signs of disintegration of the contrast fluid, the possibility of 'false' images in this examination can be ignored.

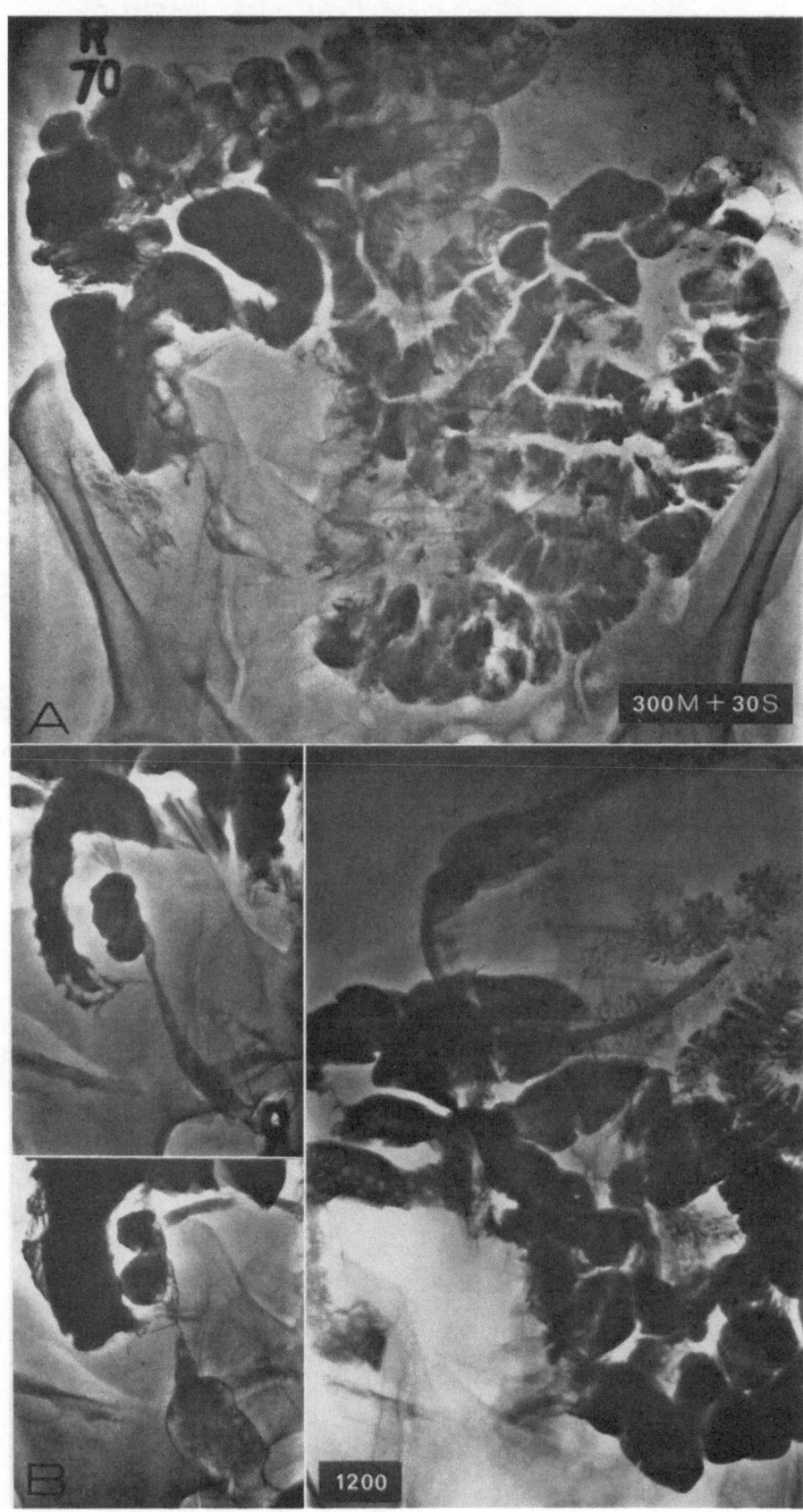

Fig. 45
Pat. 13; Infiltration in right
lower abdomen.
A: conv; 300 ml Micropaque
    + 30 g Sorbitol orally.
B: inf; 2 weeks later. 1200 ml
    Micropaque. Examination
    time 40 minutes. (Heavy
    reflux into stomach).

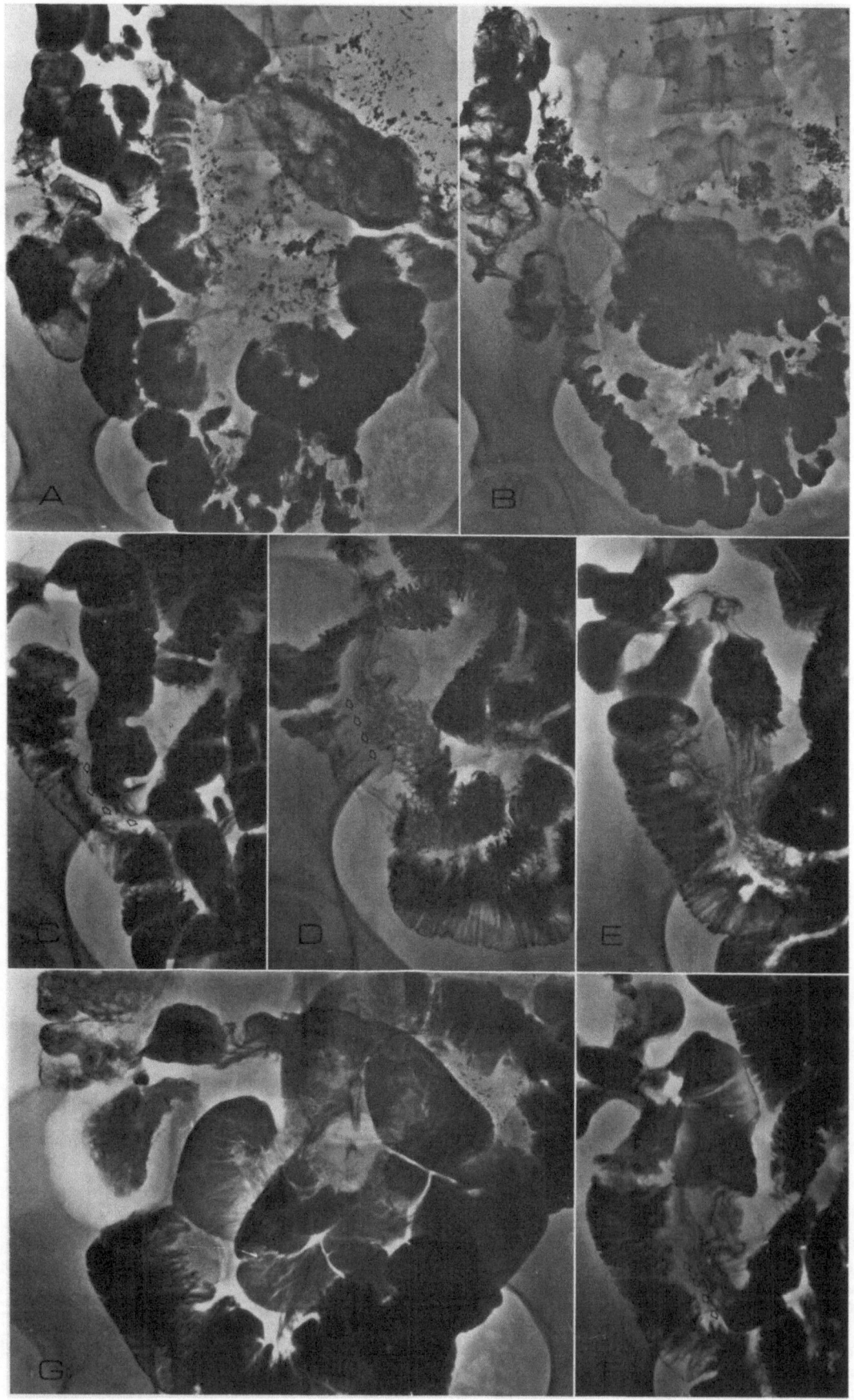

Patient 15 had an inflammation process with abscess formation in the region of the sigmoid with fistulization toward the vagina (fig. 47B). The examination after duodenal intubation showed only adhesions in the nearby loops of the small intestine (fig. 47A).

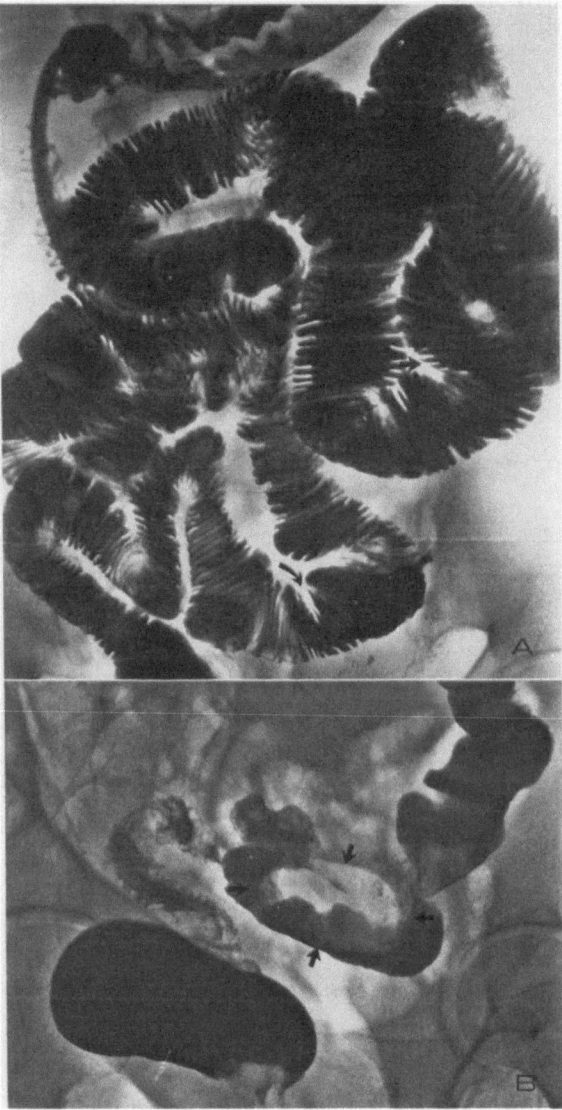

Fig 47
Pat. 15: Sigmoido-vaginal fistulous tract.
A: inf; 600 ml Microbar AZL. Adhesions on loops of small intestine.
B: infiltration with abscess formation of unknown origin in the region of the sigmoid (colon examination).

Fig. 46
Pat. 14: Abdominal complaints. Para-rectal fistulous tracts.
A, B: conventional examination 2 years ago lasted 6 hours and showed flocculation and segmentation of the contrast fluid.
C, D, E, F: dubious local abnormalities of the mucosa in the ileum. Examination after duodenal intubation with 600 ml Micropaque (s.g. 1.38) + 400 ml water. Total examination time 20 min.
G: infusion examination two months later shows no definite abnormalities; region of the valve of Bauhin is also free of abnormalities.

In *patient 16* an anomaly of the position of the cecum and appendix was observed which was at least as clearly seen on the colon examination 2 weeks previously (fig. 48B). A presumed appendicular infiltration could not be demonstrated; in particular, the flattened fold relief of the last ileum loop and the wide space between this loop and the cecum, both seen on the double-contrast exposures made during the colon examination, were no longer clearly visible (fig. 48A).

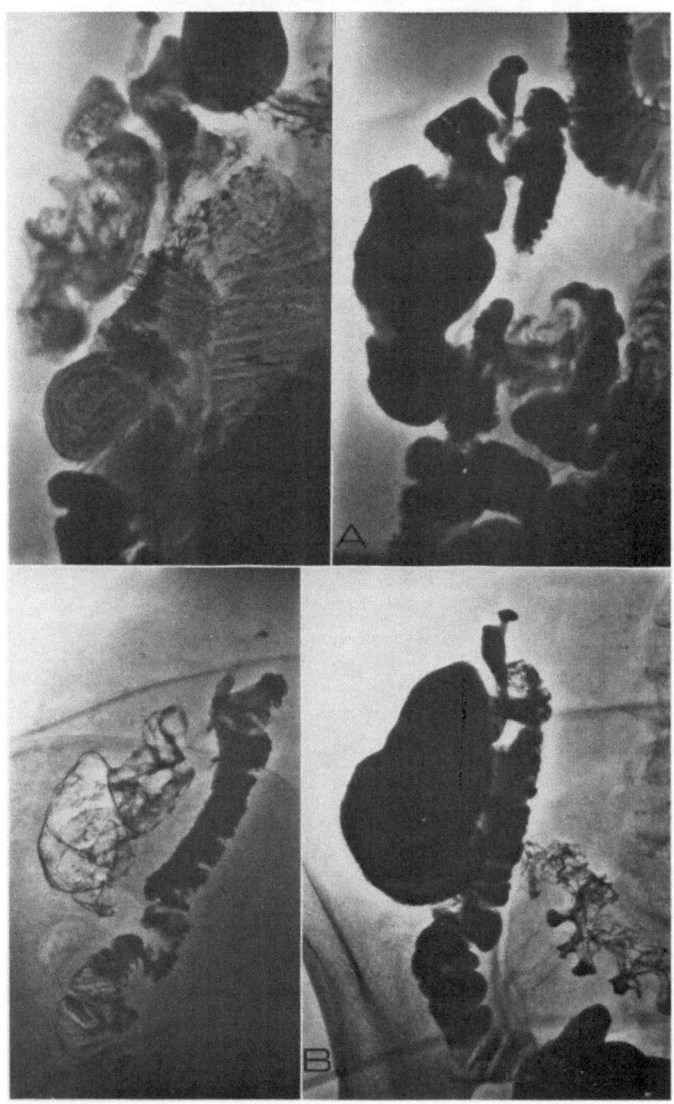

Fig. 48
Pat. 16: Abdominal complaints.
A: inf; 600 ml Microbar AZL (s.g. 1.65) followed by 600 ml water.
   Anomaly of position of cecum and appendix. No definite ab-
   normality of last ileal loop.
B: colon; 2 weeks previously. Wide space between ileum and cecum;
   flattening of fold relief. Inflammation process close by?

IV

Seventeen patients were examined because of diarrhea or steatorrhea; the causes were varied and in some cases unknown. Anatomical abnormalities were found in only two of these patients.

Patient 17 was an obese 63-year-old man who had complained lately of severe diarrhea. The results of the radiological examination conflicted entirely with the short history. Extensive abnormalities were found in the ileum which must be ascribed to Crohn's disease (fig. 49).

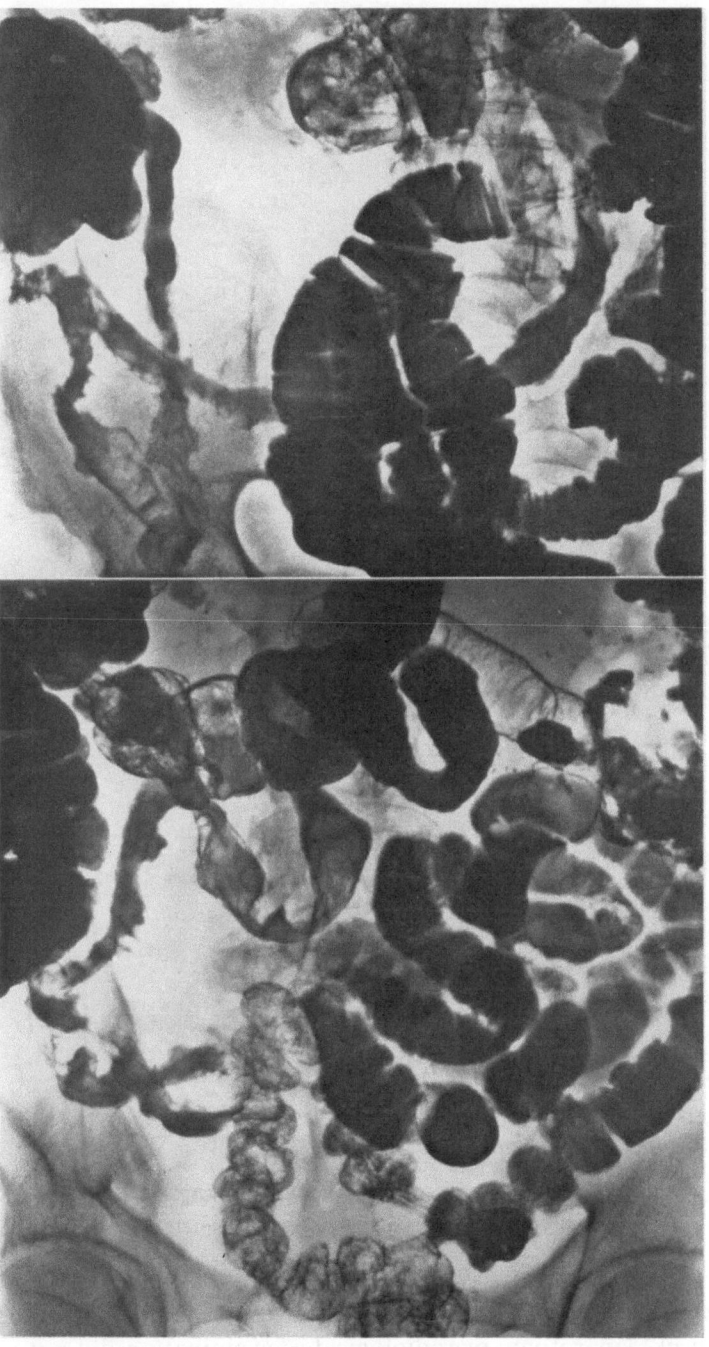

Fig. 49
Pat. 17: Vague abdominal complaints.
inf; 1200 ml barium suspension (s.g. 1.28).
Extensive abnormalities in ileum. Crohn's disease.

Patient 18 was a 51-year-old female. For the past 6 months she had suffered from an irregular but severe steatorrhea. The duodenal infusion technique revealed local abnormalities of the ileum in the right lower abdomen; interpretation was difficult (fig. 50B). Probably there were adhesions, narrowing of the intestinal lumen and thickening of the intestinal wall. The conventional examination 4 months earlier revealed no abnormalities; however the ileum loop in question was not filled during this

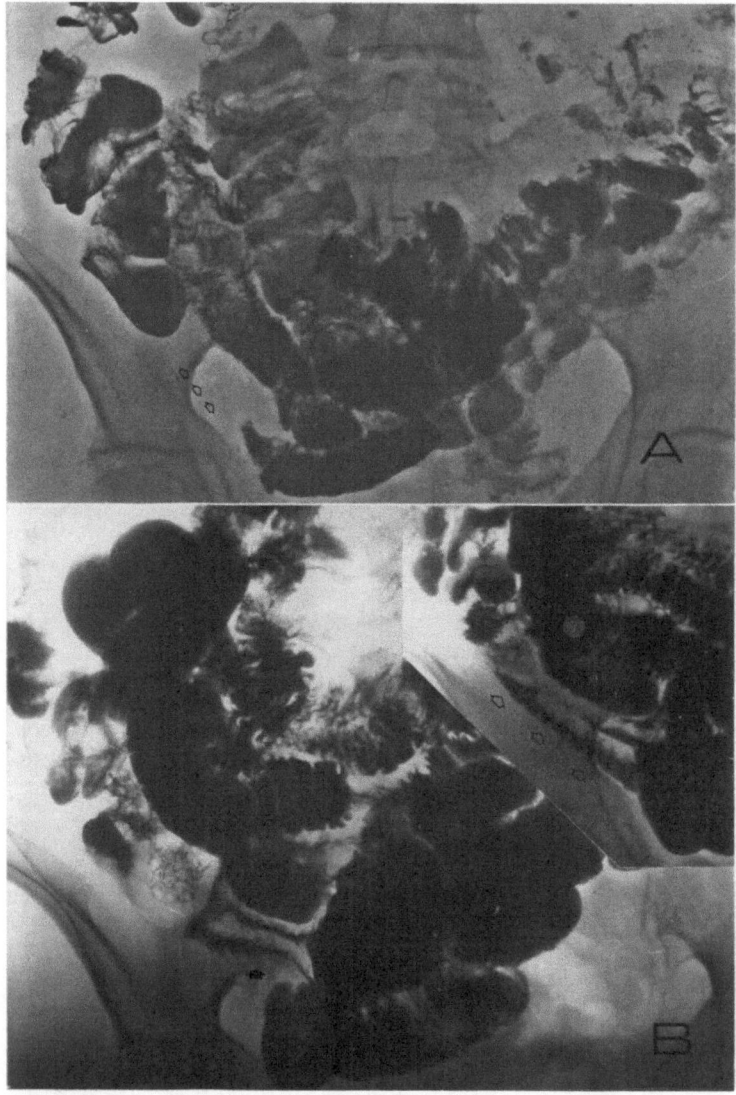

Fig. 50
Pat. 18: Severe steatorrhea.
A: conv. examination.
B: 4 months later, 600 ml contrast fluid through tube. Abnormalities of
   unknown nature in right lower abdomen. Adequate compression not
   possible.

examination (fig. 50A). Since several weeks later metastases of an adenocarcinoma were found in the lymph glands of the neck, laparotomy or radiological re-examination did not occur.

Four other patients of this group had also been examined previously by the conventional method; two less than 2 months ago and two 8 and 10 months ago. The x-rays from the conventional examination of these 4 patients all showed heavy flocculation and segmentation of the contrast fluid so that anatomical evaluation was impossible. For this reason, we consider the discussion of these patients especially important. In spite of the fact that large dosages of stable contrast fluid and enhancement of gastric emptying have resulted in great improvement, these patients belong in a category for which conventional examination techniques often yield no anatomical information at all.

These 4 patients were examined using the duodenal infusion technique; only *patient 19*, who had a severe steatorrhea, showed flocculation of the contrast medium in such an early stage that anatomical information of the ileum could no longer be obtained (fig. 51). The flocculation in this patient was facilitated by the following factors:

1. As contrast medium, the relatively unstable Microbar AZL was used.
2. 600 ml contrast medium was considered a sufficient dose.
3. Since this was one of our first patients, the infusion period was rather long (10 min.).

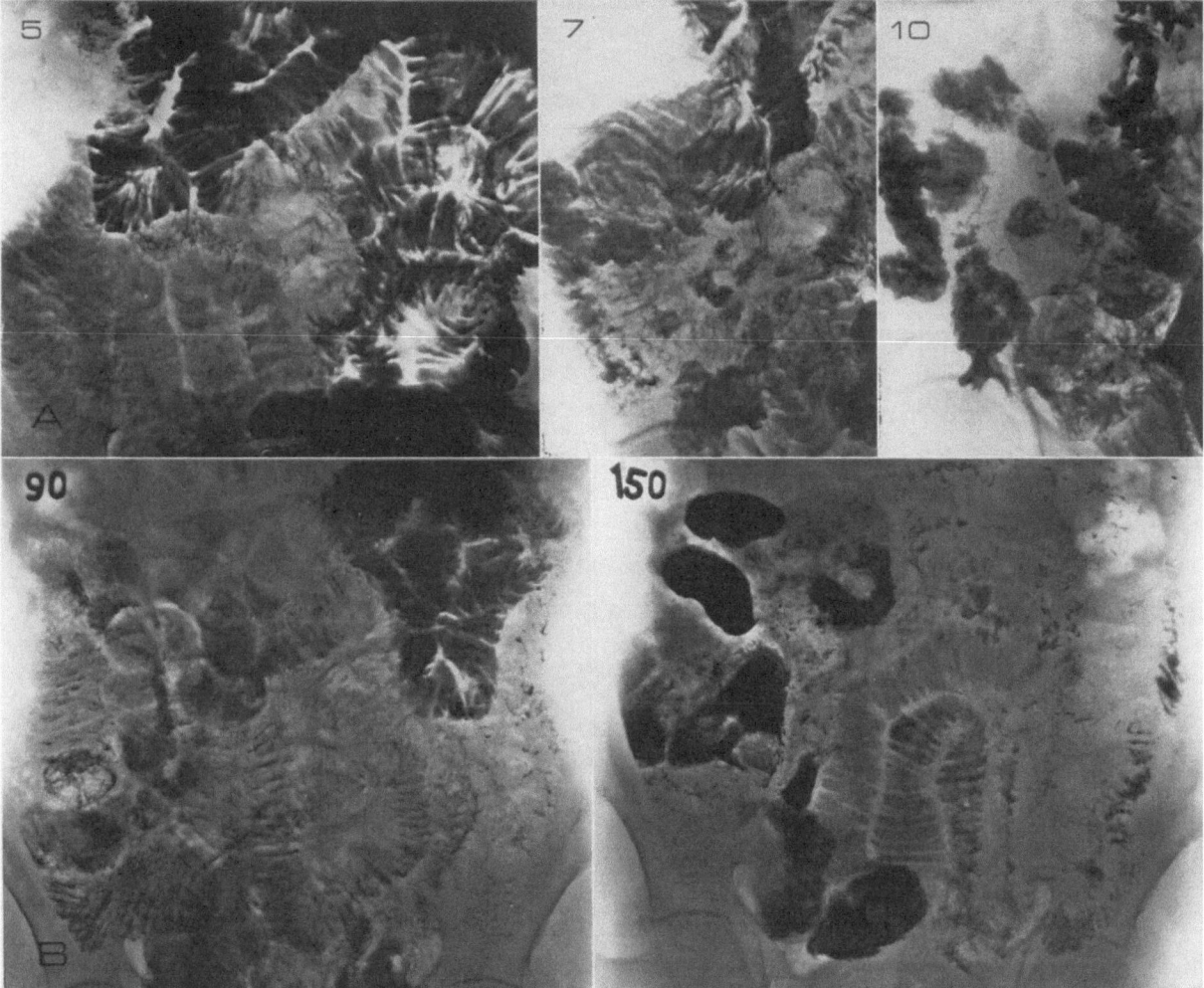

Fig. 51
Pat. 19: severe steatorrhea.
A: 600 ml Microbar AZL administered through tube in 10 minutes. Five and 7 minutes later, useful exposures of jejunum in left half of abdomen. Rapidly increasing disintegration in right half of abdomen.
B: 8 weeks later, 300 ml Microbar AZL orally.

The x-rays obtained using the infusion technique clearly provide more information than those obtained by the conventional radiological technique for *patient 20* (cellulose allergy), *patient 21* (gluten-sensitive sprue) and *patient 22* (figs. 52, 53 and 54). The conventional transit examination of patient 20 took place only 3 weeks previously; 300 ml Micropaque with 30 ml Solcoray was administered. For the examination after duodenal intubation, 600 ml of the same contrast medium was used without Solcoray.

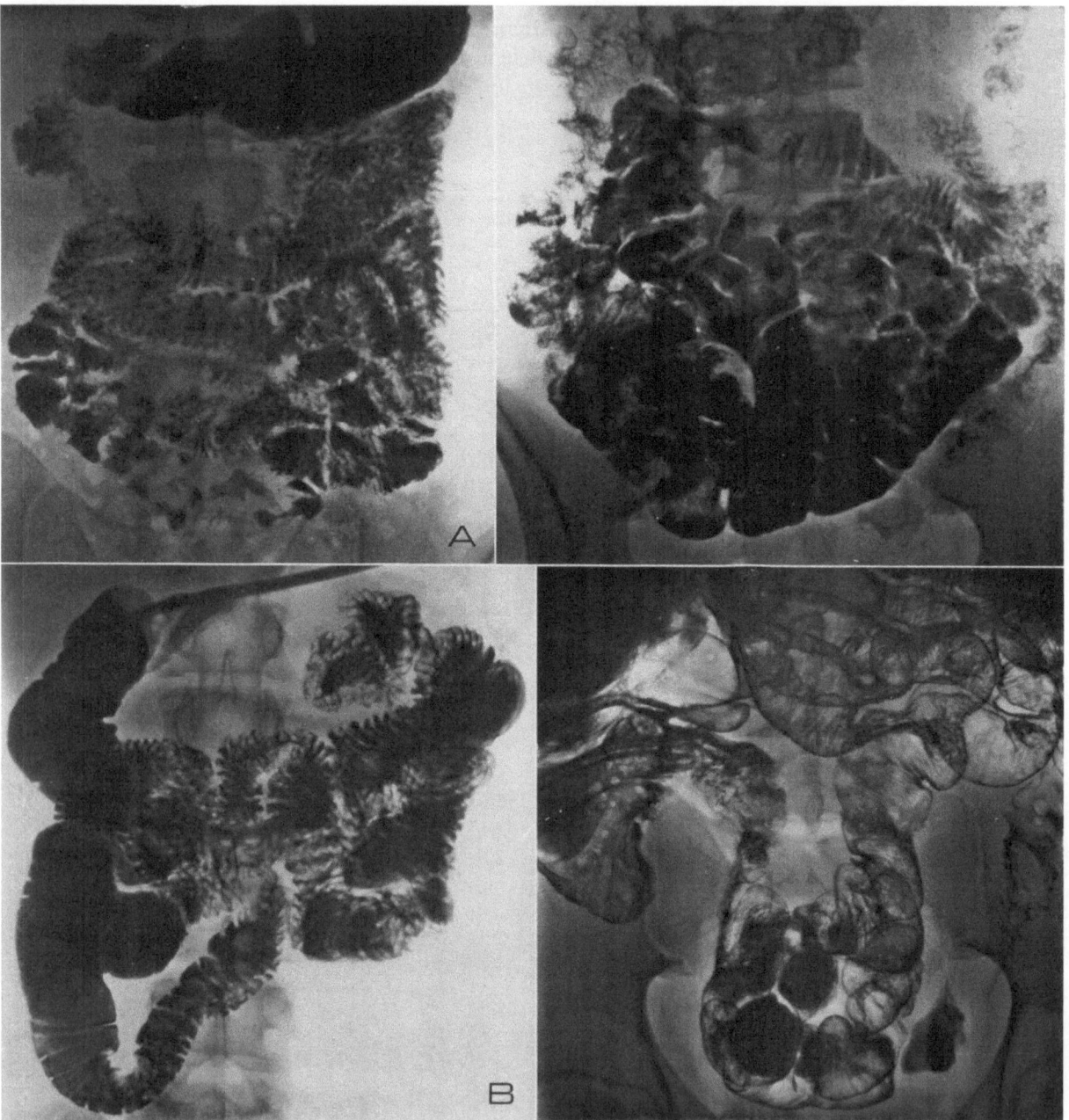

Fig. 52
Pat. 20: cellulose allergy.
A: conv; 300 ml Micropaque + 30 ml Solcoray.
B, C: inf; 3 weeks later, 600 ml Micropaque + air insufflation. Good mucosal patterns in jejunum and ileum.

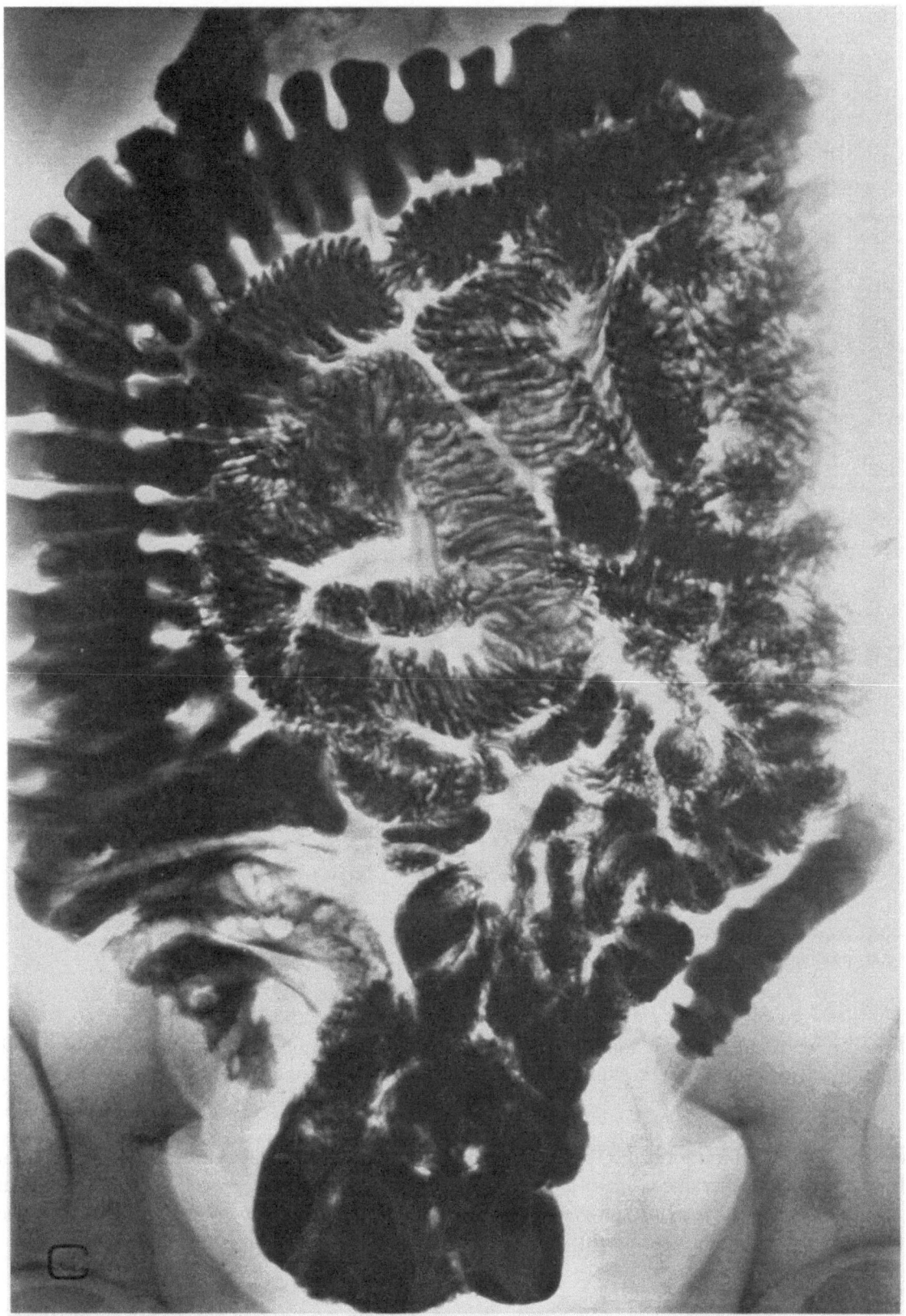

Fig. 52c

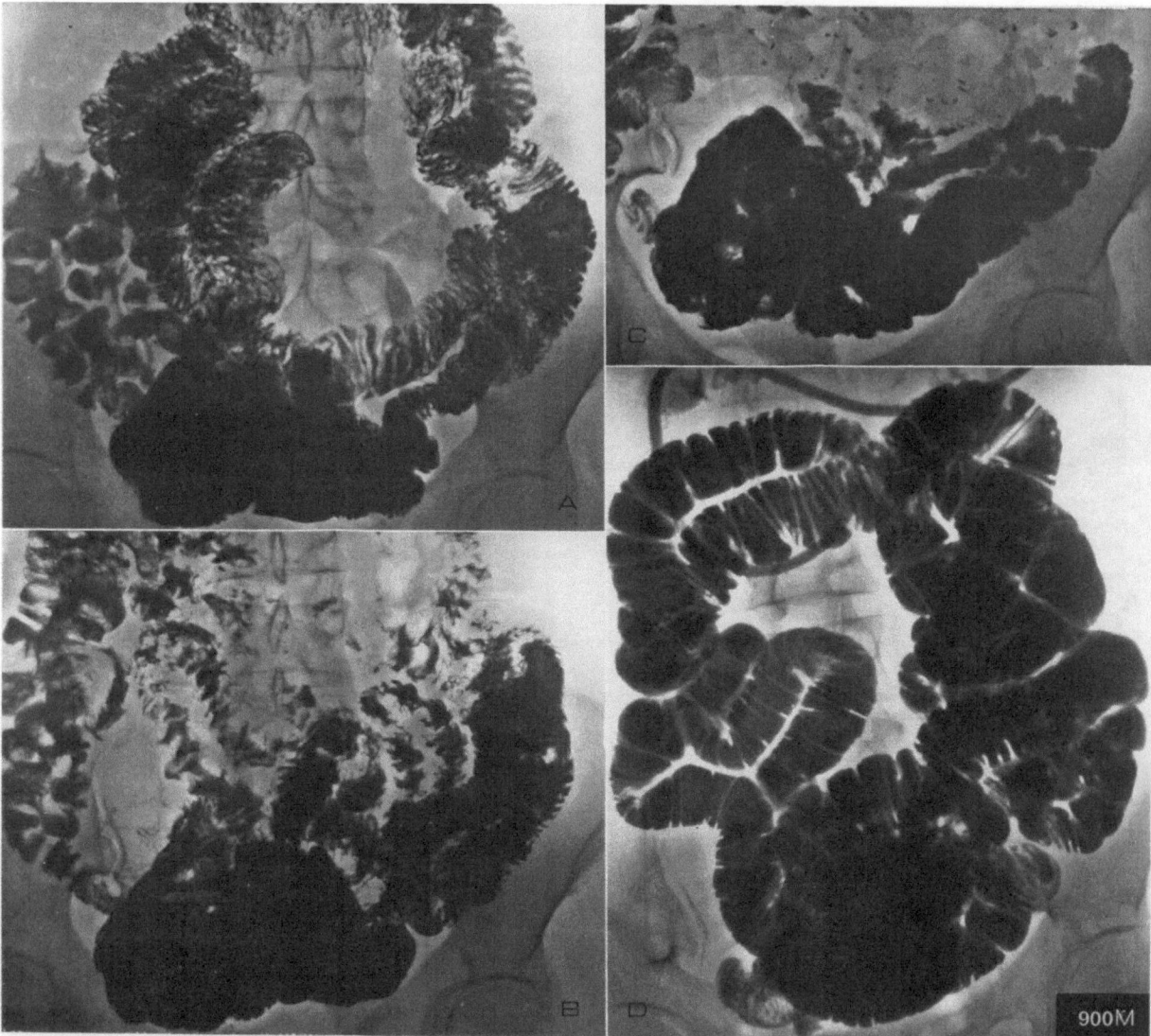

Fig. 53
Pat. 21: gluten-sensitive sprue.
A, B, C: conv. examination.

In *patient 23*, who had not been examined by the conventional technique, an early flocculation of the contrast fluid also occurred. The films of the jejunum and ileum had however already been made (fig. 55).

The average total examination time for the 17 patients in this group was 33 minutes and therefore slightly less than the general average of 36 minutes. However a complete as well as excellent barium filling of the colon and rectosigmoid was seen so often that we have come to believe that the intensified peristalsis related to diarrhea is more frequently located in the colon than in the small intestine.

V

Five patients were examined because of rectal blood loss and no abnormalities of the small intestine were found. None of these 5 patients had had a previous conventional transit examination.

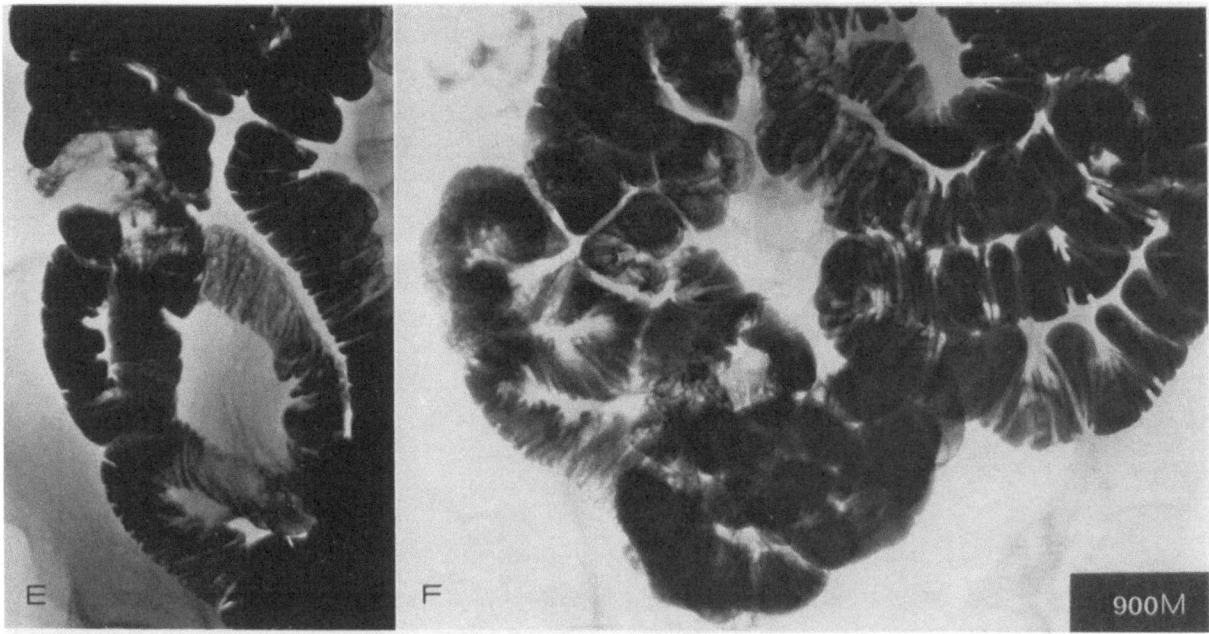

Fig. 53

D, E, F: 8 months later, 900 Micr. AZL through tube. Good pictures of entire small intestine, no disintegration of contrast fluid.

VI

Patient 24 underwent an examination of the small intestine because of the development of fever of unknown origin. With the exception of one adhesion, no abnormalities were found (fig. 56). A conventional examination did not take place.

VII

Four patients had been treated for a malignant tumor of the internal genitalia by irradiation of the abdominal area. A conventional transit examination had not been carried out for any of these patients. For one patient the examination had been requested because a portion of the ileum was to be used as the new bladder. A second patient was examined for back pain. Neither of these patients had complaints relating to the digestive tract and no abnormalities were found.

The other two patients did have intestinal symptoms, consisting mainly of painful cramps and diarrhea. In *patient 25* only a very active peristalsis was observed in the small intestine and in the colon a stricture was found. The x-rays of *patient 26* showed a large process in the left lower abdomen. Multiple adhesions can be seen, as well as a number of intestinal loops with obviously thickened walls probably due to lymphedema (fig. 57).

VIII

Of 8 patients, 7 were examined after duodenal intubation because of symptoms apparently caused by a stenosis in the small intestine.

The eighth patient (*patient 27*) had a routine examination because a jejunal tumor had been removed two years previously. No recurrence of the tumor was seen; due to an increase in the fluid supply during the examination, the location of the anastomosis could be seen clearly (fig. 58).

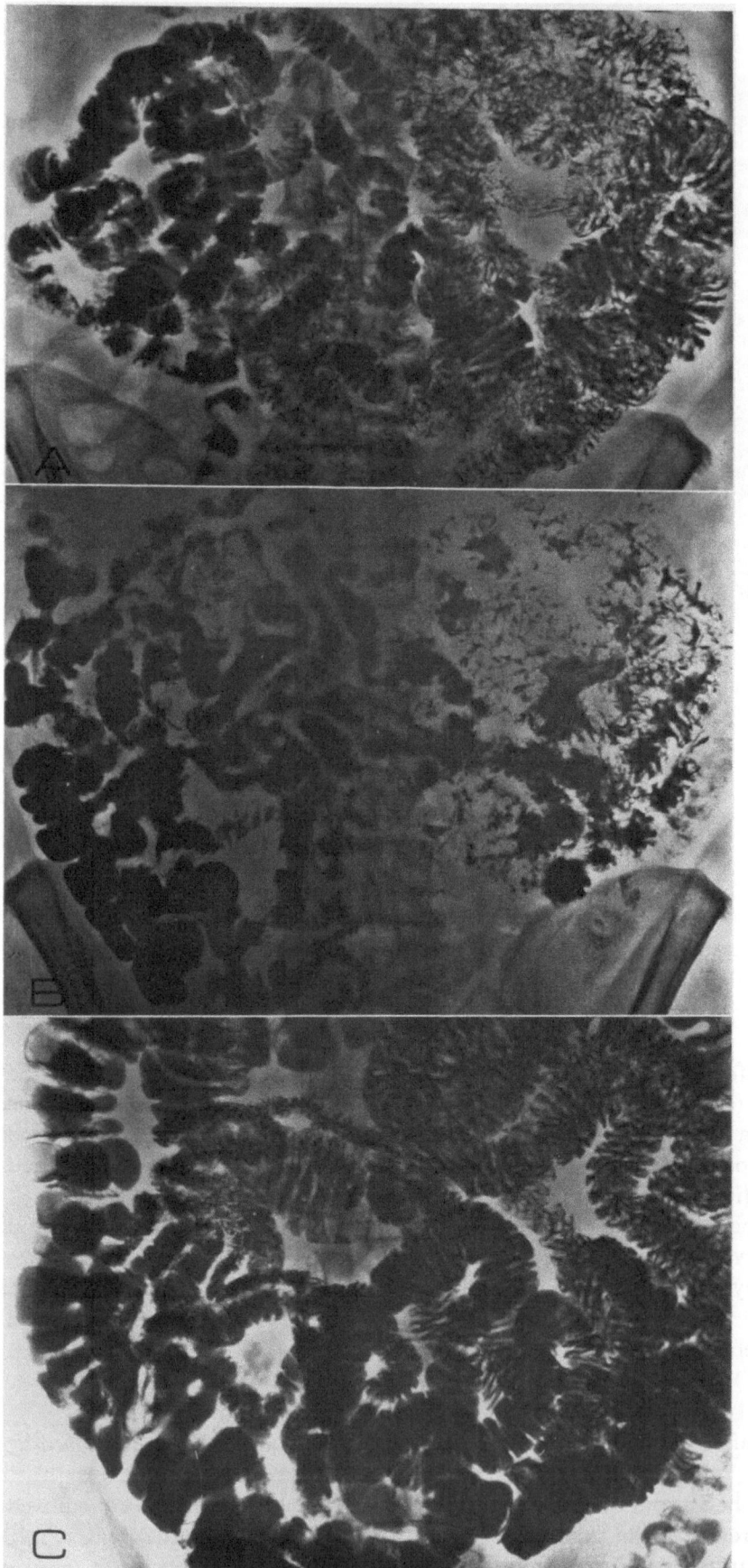

Fig. 54
Pat. 22: malabsorption of unknown origin.
A, B: conv. examination, 300 ml Micr. AZL orally.
C: 11 months later, 1000 ml Mixobar through tube in 20 min. Position of ileum loops quite clear.

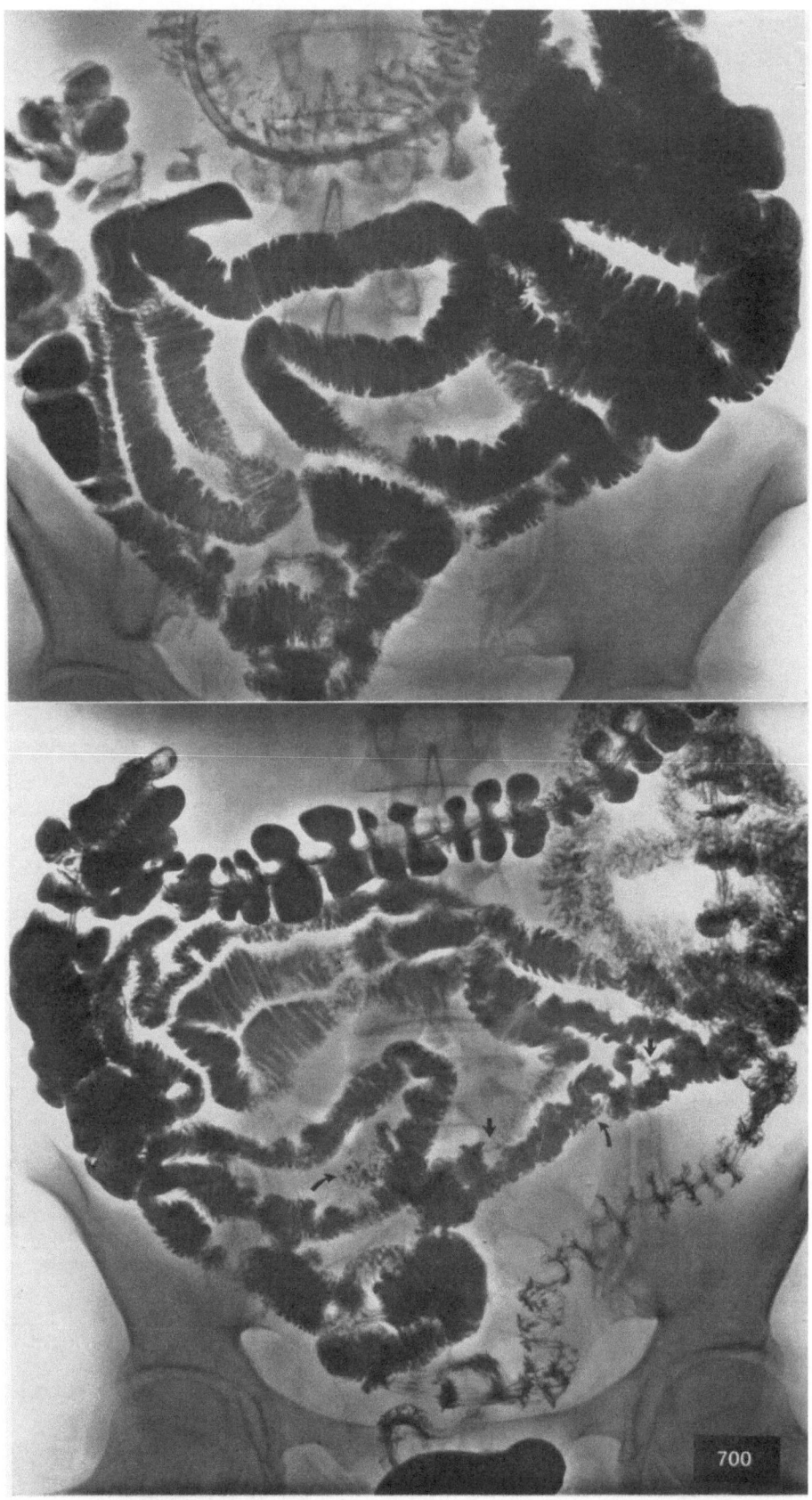

Fig. 55
Pat. 23; diarrhea of unknown origin.
700 ml Micr. AZL through tube. Position of ileum loops very clear. Last exposure shows beginning flocculation of contrast fluid.

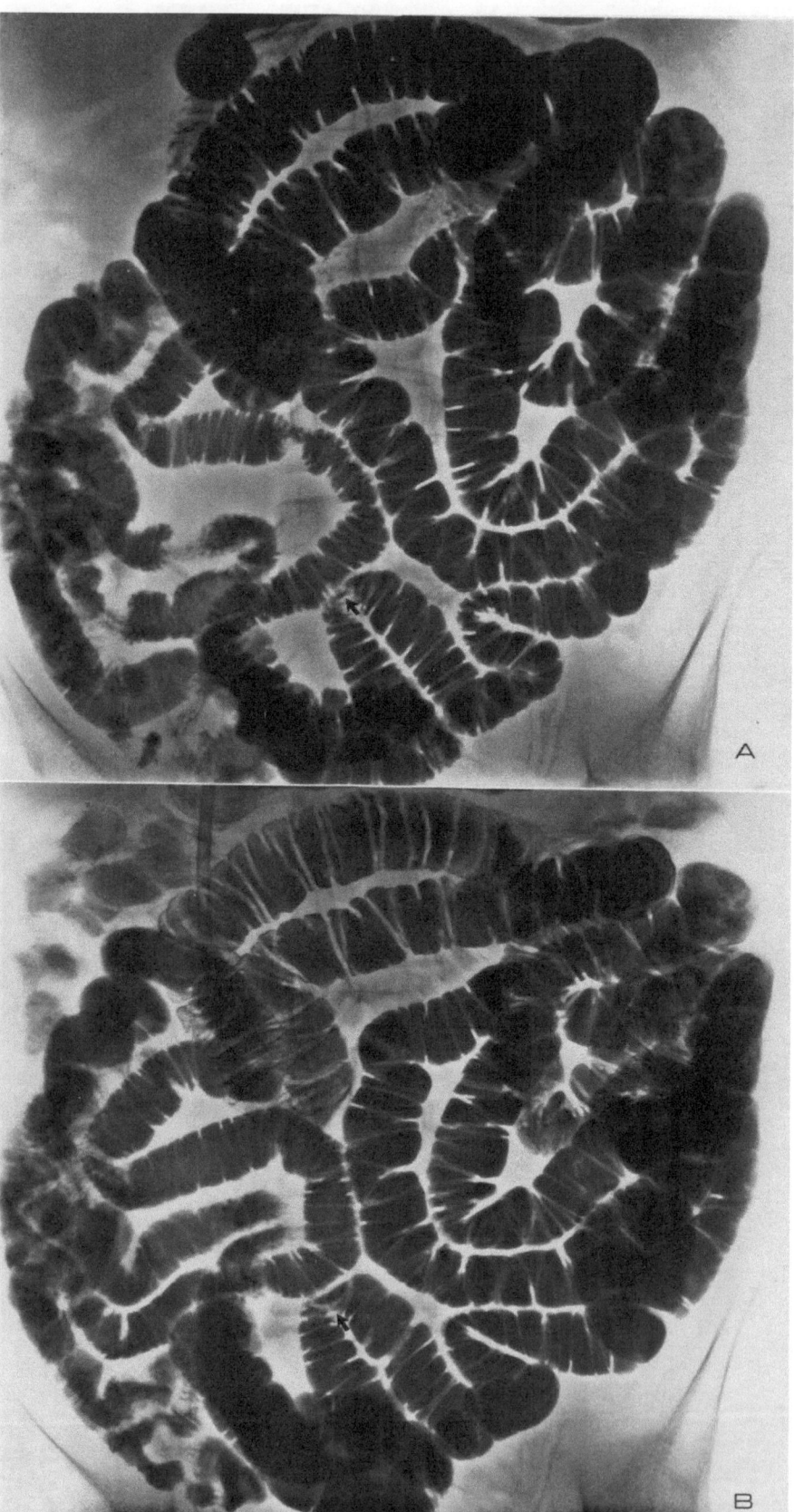

Fig. 56
Pat. 24: fever of unknown
origin.
1200 ml barium suspension
(s.g. 1.27) administered
through tube in 10 min.,
followed by 600 ml water and
oral air insufflation. Local
adhesion of 2 ileum loops, no
further abnormalities.
Position of intestinal loops
quite clear in this
pronounced pycnic.

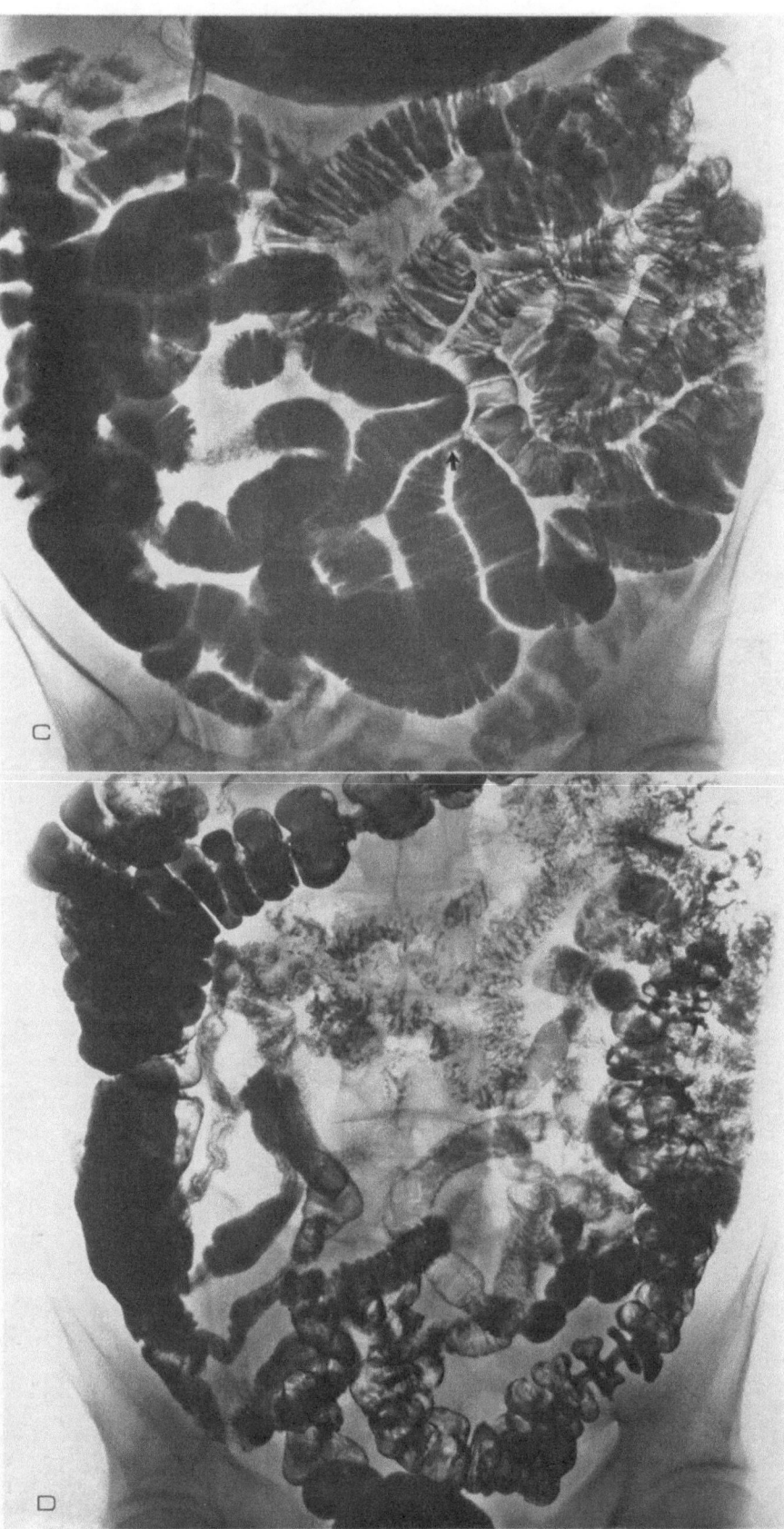

Fig. 56
continued

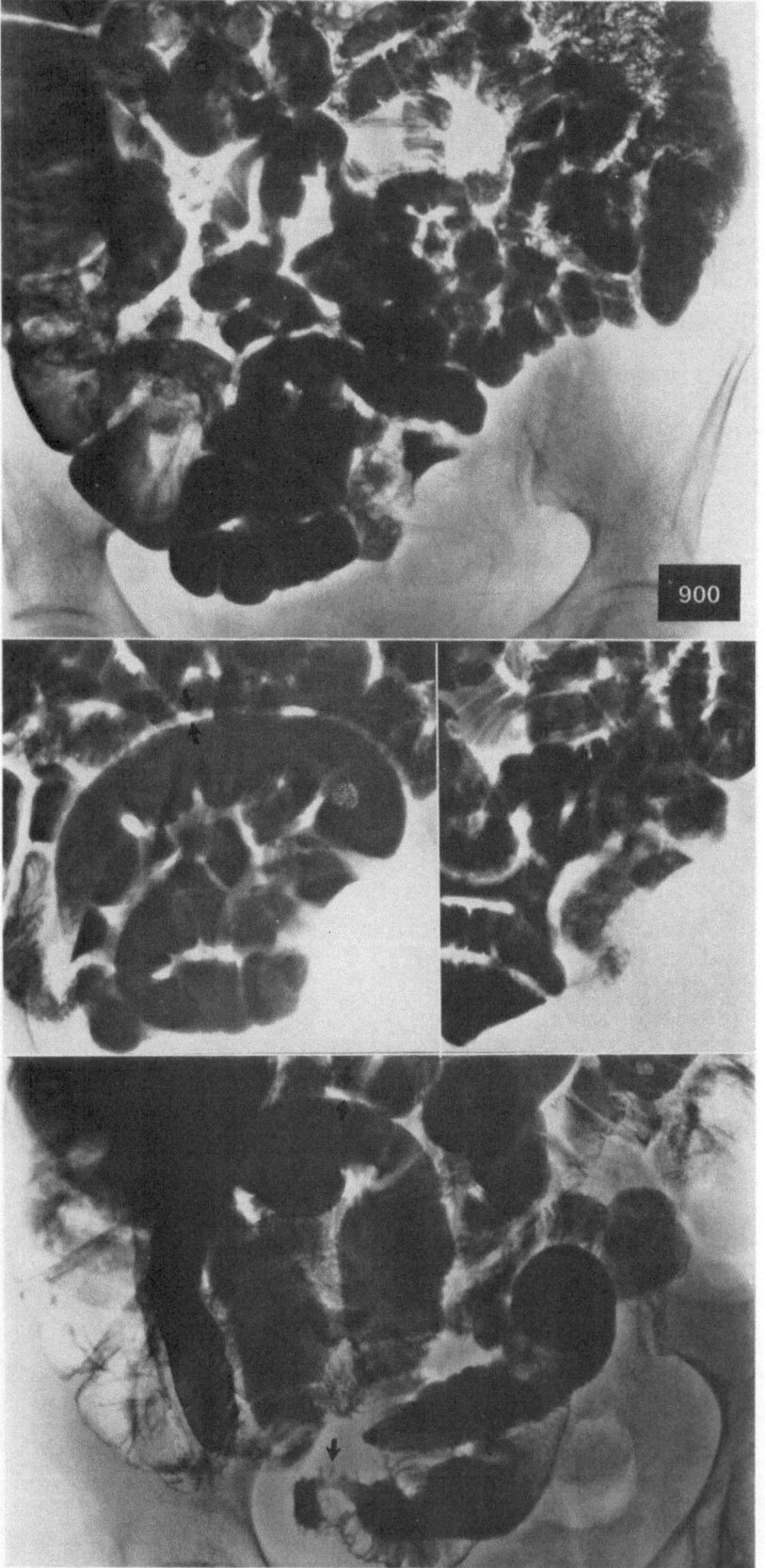

Fig. 57
Pat. 26: two years ago 6000 R TD in
region of small pelvis because of
cervix carc.
Now painful cramps and diarrhea.
Infusion of 900 ml Micr. AZL.
Compression not feasible. Large
process in left lower abdomen.
Adhesions and obviously thickened
intestinal walls.

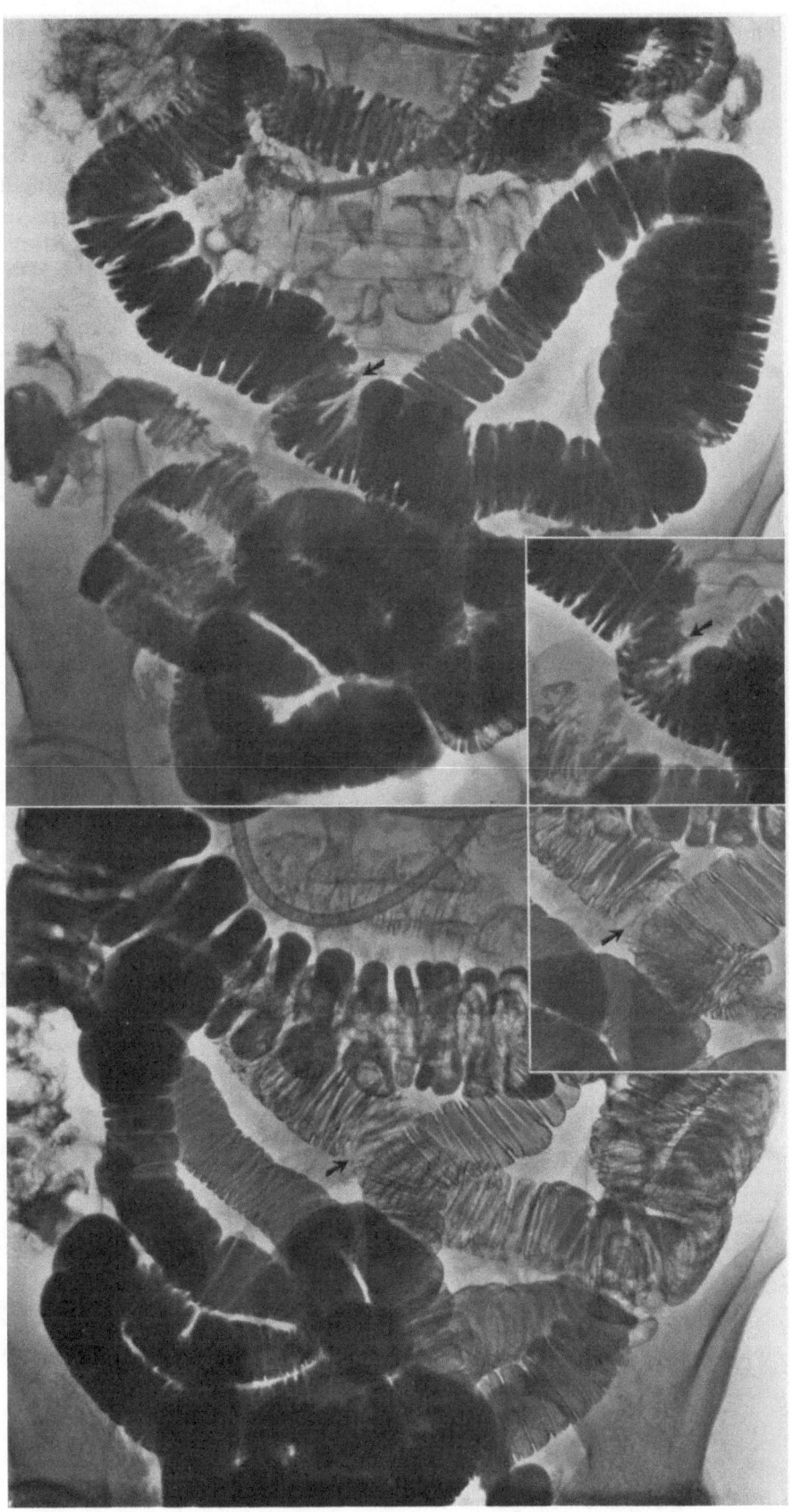

Fig. 58
Pat. 27: jejunal tumor removed
2 years ago. Control examination, no complaints.
600 ml Micropaque (s.g. 1.26)
through tube followed by
600 ml water 5 minutes later.
No recurrence, relative
narrowing of anastomosis
clearly seen.

Only one of these 8 patients had been examined (elsewhere) by the conventional method and no abnormalities were found; the colon examination also revealed nothing (*patient 28*, figs. 59A, B). The infusion examination several months later showed an egg-sized polypoid mass in the cecum; during surgery it was seen that this mass originated from the mucosa (figs. 59C, D).

The radiological examination of 3 of the remaining 6 patients also showed abnormalities.
Patient 29 had had 2 ileum resections because of extensive strangulations and adhesions. Here adhesions are seen once again between the ileal loops in the small pelvis (figs. 60, 61).

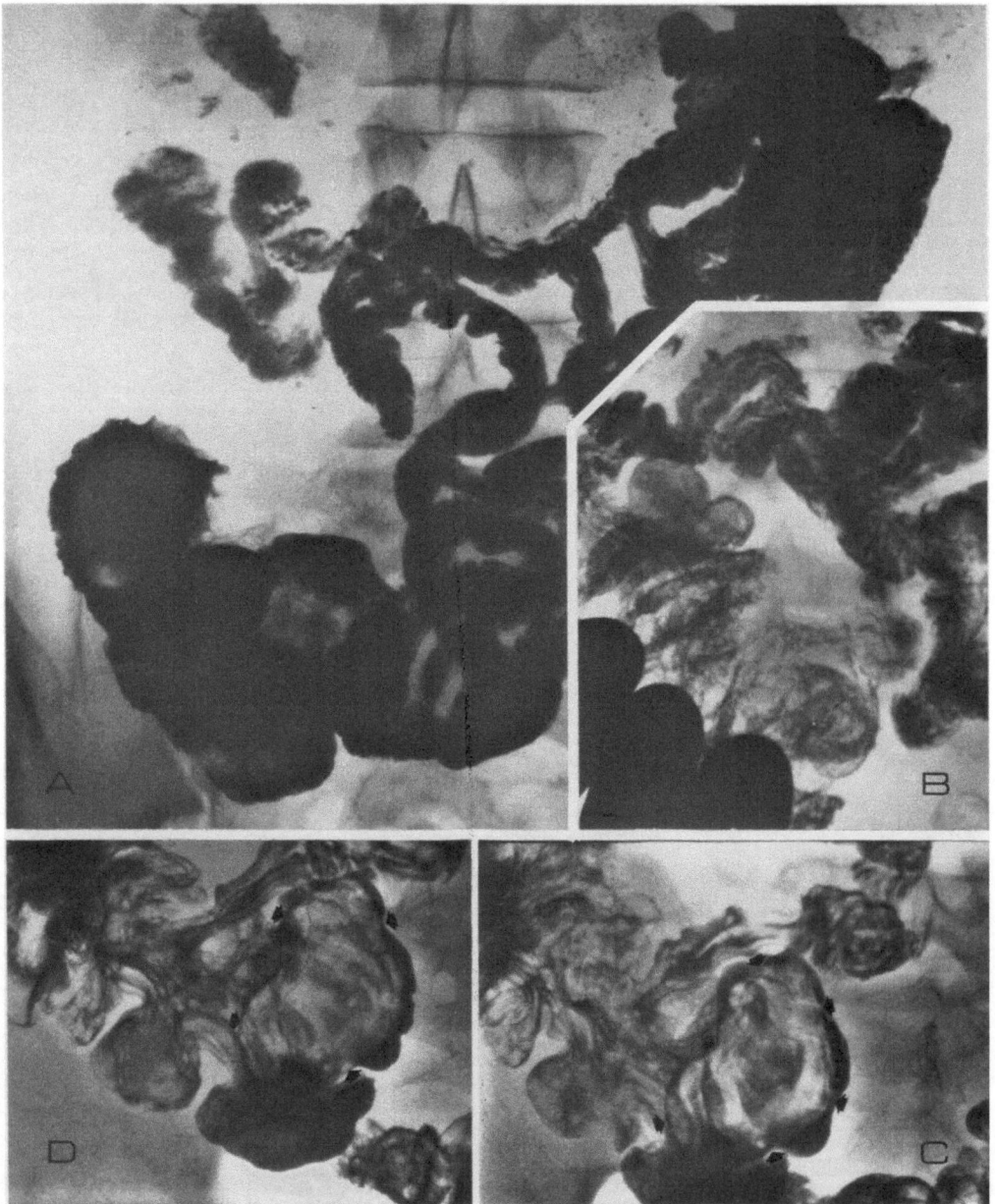

Fig. 59
Pat. 28: periodic attacks of severe abdominal pains over past few years.
A: conv. transit examination, no abnormalities.
B: colon examination, no abnormalities.
C, D: 3 months later, after duodenal intubation, large polypoid mass seen in cecum. Surgical findings show that mass originated from mucosa.

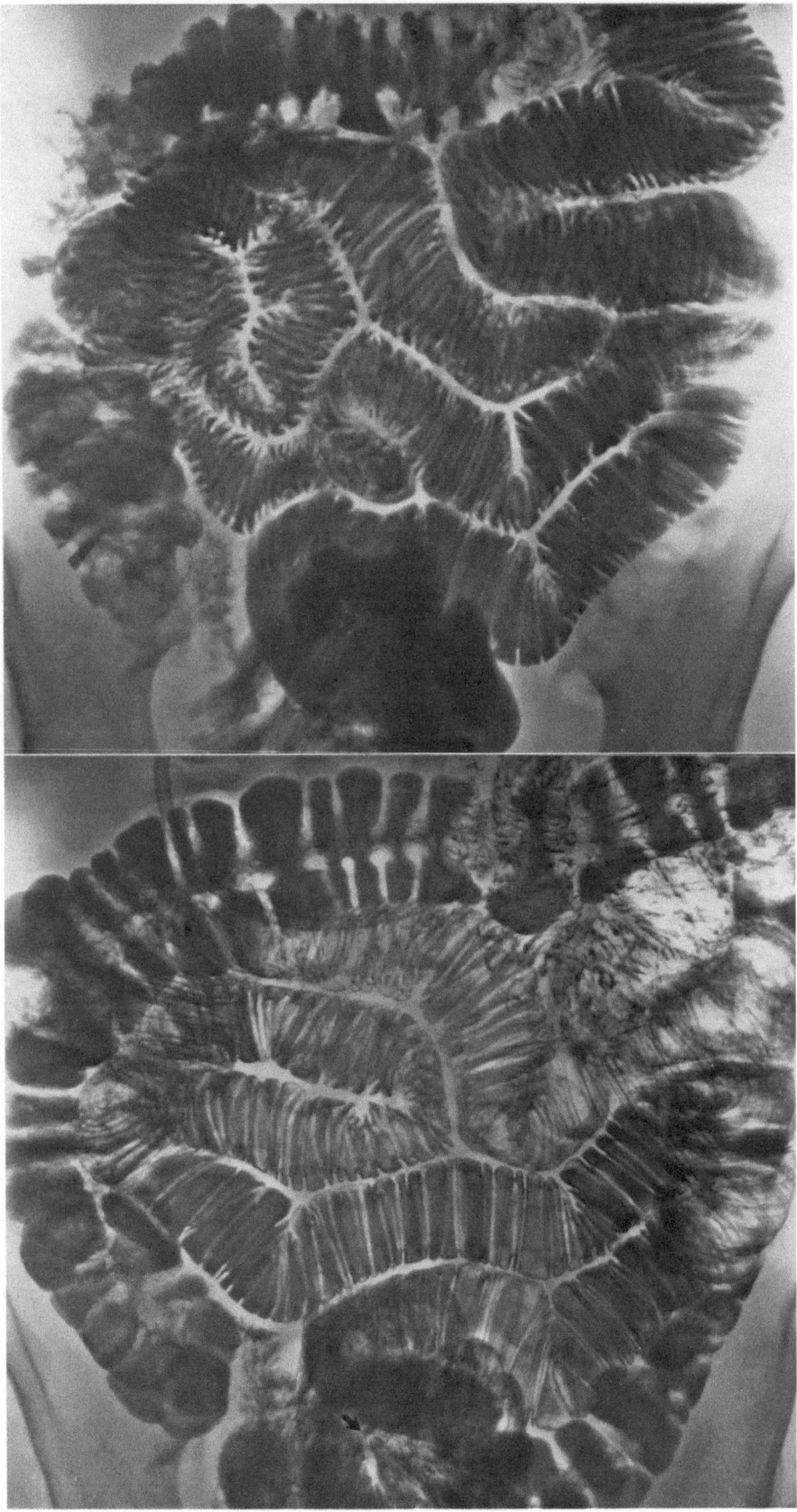

Fig. 60
Pat. 29: periodic symptoms of
ileus. In the past 2 partial
ileum resections because of
strangulation.
Infusion examination: 750 ml
barium suspension (s.g. 1.2)
followed by oral air
insufflation. Mass of ileum
loops in small pelvis.
Adhesions.

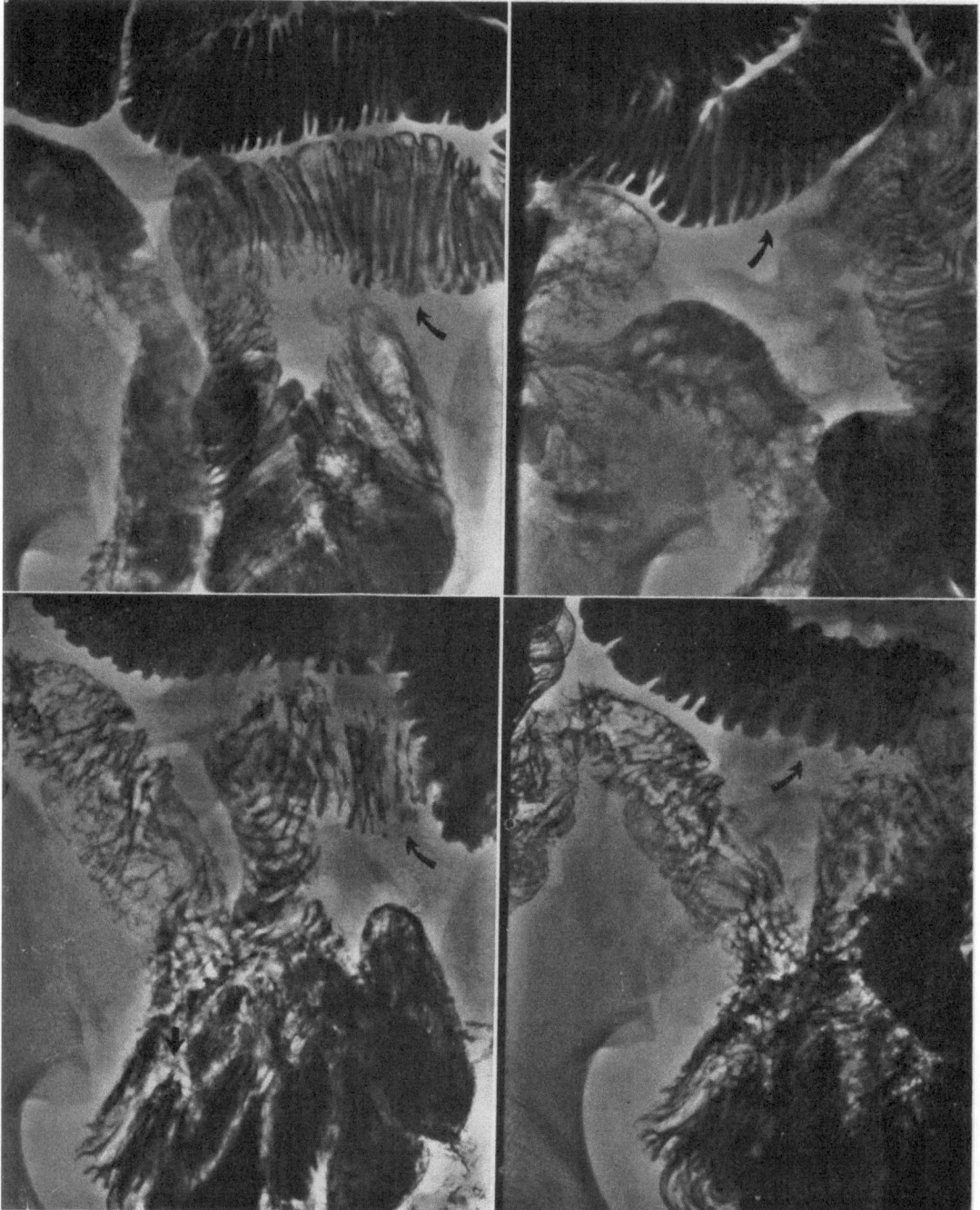

Fig. 61
Pat. 29: On the 2 uppermost exposures the mucosal folds appear normal; disintegration of the contrast fluid
then developed rapidly with flattening and apparent coarsening of the mucosal folds (2 lowermost exposures).
The structure of the contrast fluid has become granular.

In *patient 30* a stenosis, thought to be a tumor, was found in the jejunum which surgical and pathological examination proved to be due to adenocarcinoma (fig. 62). The x-rays clearly showed that
marked prestenotic dilatation developed due to an increase in fluid supply.

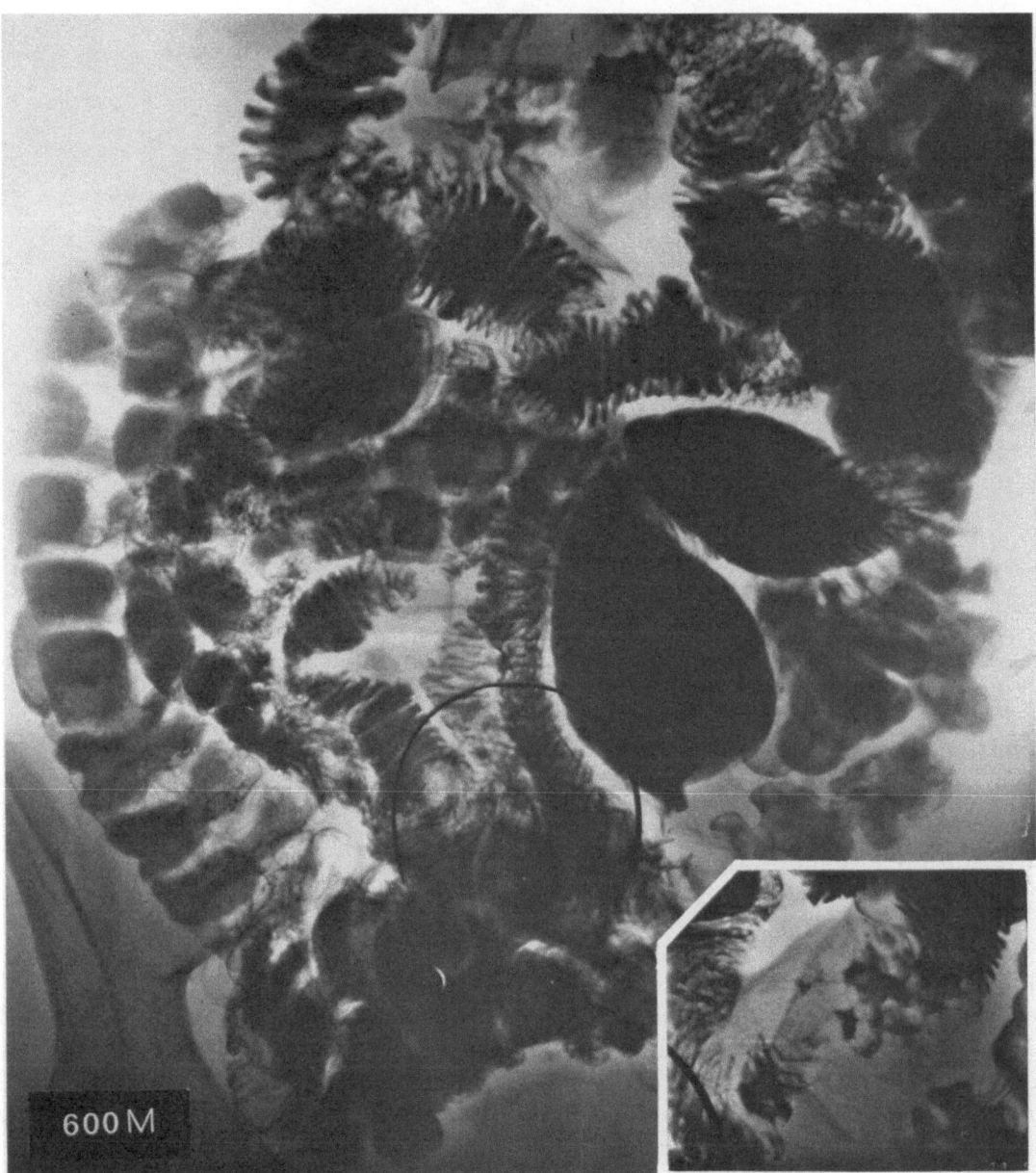

600 M

Fig. 62
Pat. 30: adenocarcinoma of the jejunum.
Prestenotic dilatation by rapid fluid supply (600 ml in 10 min.).

Patient 31 was a 70-year-old male admitted because of an acute proximal ileus. Invagination, volvulus or a vascular accident were considered. The film made immediately after 600 ml contrast fluid (300 ml Micropaque + 300 ml water) was administered through a tube, shows very wide jejunal loops (fig. 63). The cecum had not yet been reached on this exposure and the location of the obstruction cannot yet be seen. Periods of active peristalsis alternating with aperistalsis were observed. Fifteen minutes later it was decided to administer a slightly diluted second dose of 600 ml contrast medium (200 ml Micropaque + 400 ml water).This resulted in a sudden acceleration of the previously very slow transit and the disappearance of the dilatation of the jejunal loops. On the x-rays then taken a more or less vertical intestinal loop in the mid-abdominal region was seen with a markedly swollen mucosa and a defenite thickening of the intestinal wall, as usually seen in a mesenteric thrombosis

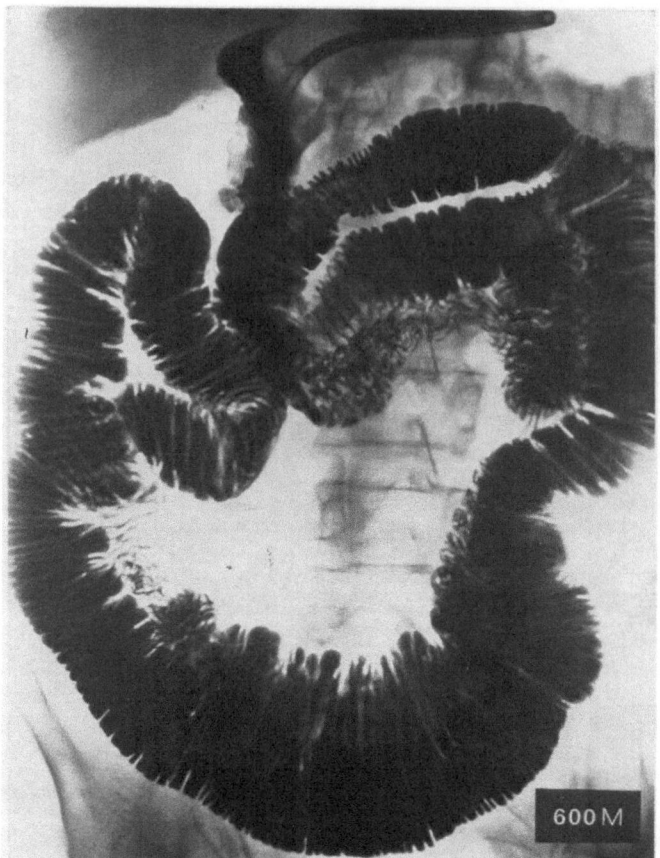

Fig. 63
Pat. 31: sudden acute proximal ileus.
Wide jejunal loops after administration of 600 ml Micropaque
through tube.

(fig. 64A). Surprisingly the patient's condition improved rapidly so that abdominal compression, not tolerated at the beginning of the examination, was now quite feasible. Since the permanence of this provisional success could not be predicted and urgent surgical intervention was still highly likely, another 600 ml water was administered in order to force the contrast fluid out of the small intestine insofar as possible. This happened without difficulty. The condition of the patient continued to improve and an operation was not necessary.

Seven weeks later, the roentgenological examination was repeated. Neither dilatation nor obstruction were seen and the cecum was reached in five minutes. It was remarkable that this examination again showed in the mid-abdominal region one jejunal loop with pronounced flattening of the normal mucosal relief extending at least 15 cm. Furthermore one section of this loop seemed to show several centimeters of moderate narrowing (fig. 64B). To judge by these two examinations, a vascular accident seems to be most likely, although the clinical symptoms do not support this diagnosis in any way, nor did an equally rapid third radiological examination 6 weeks after the second. This third set of exposures revealed no convincing abnormalities (fig. 65).

The 3 patients without abnormalities had vague or intermittent symptoms of obstruction; at the time of the radiological examination, they had no complaints.

For the 7 patients with complaints resulting from stenosis, the average examination time was longer: 45 minutes instead of 36. In addition, the average quantity of fluid and contrast fluid administered was larger: 1140 ml instead of 900 ml.

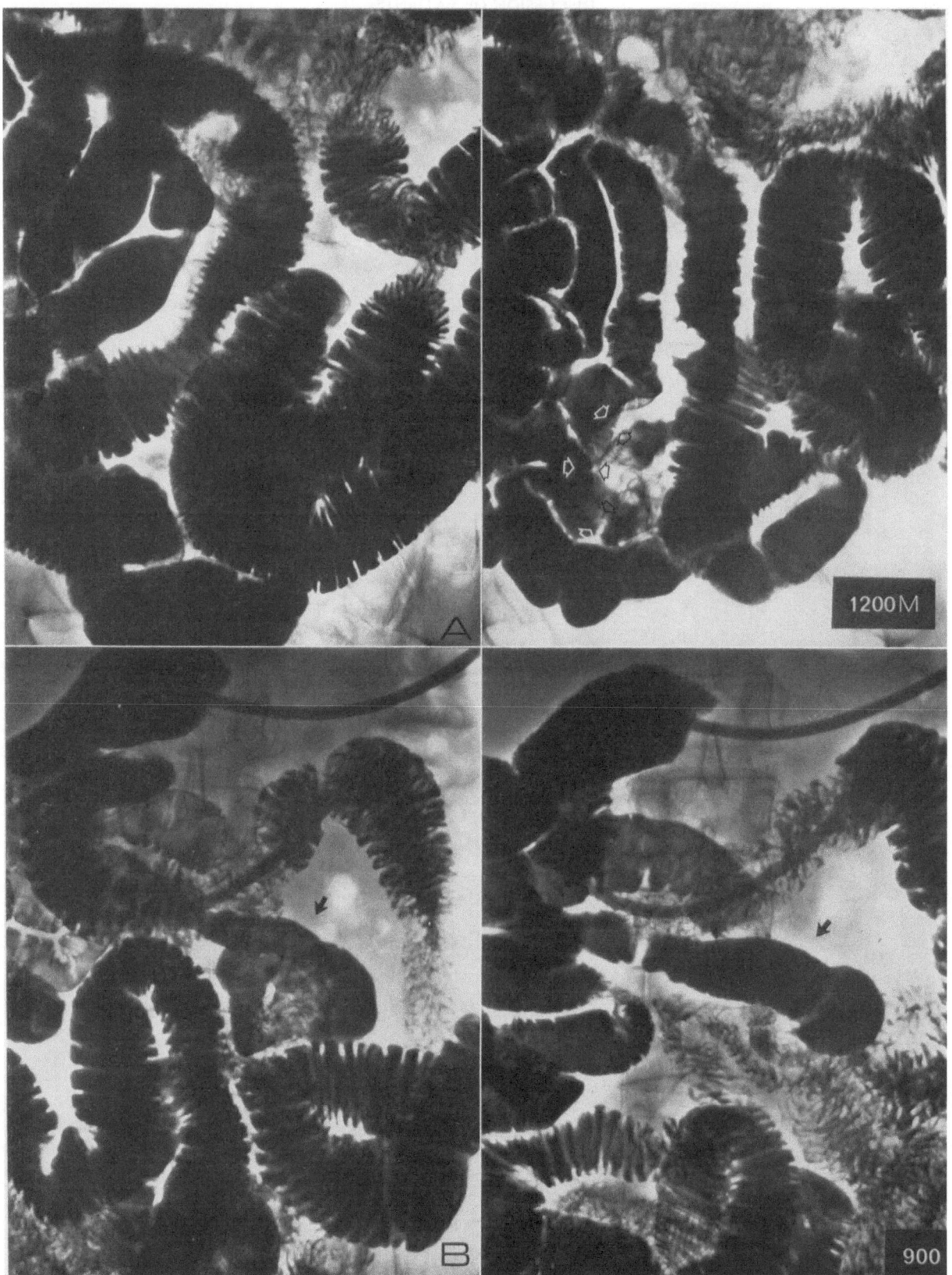

Fig. 64
Pat 31:
A: Intestinal loop with greatly thickened wall and coarse mucosal folds (1200 ml Micropaque, s.g. 1.3).
B: 7 weeks later, 900 ml Micr. AZL (s.g. 1.32) through tube. Flattening of fold relief and decreased dilatation of one single
   jejunal loop.

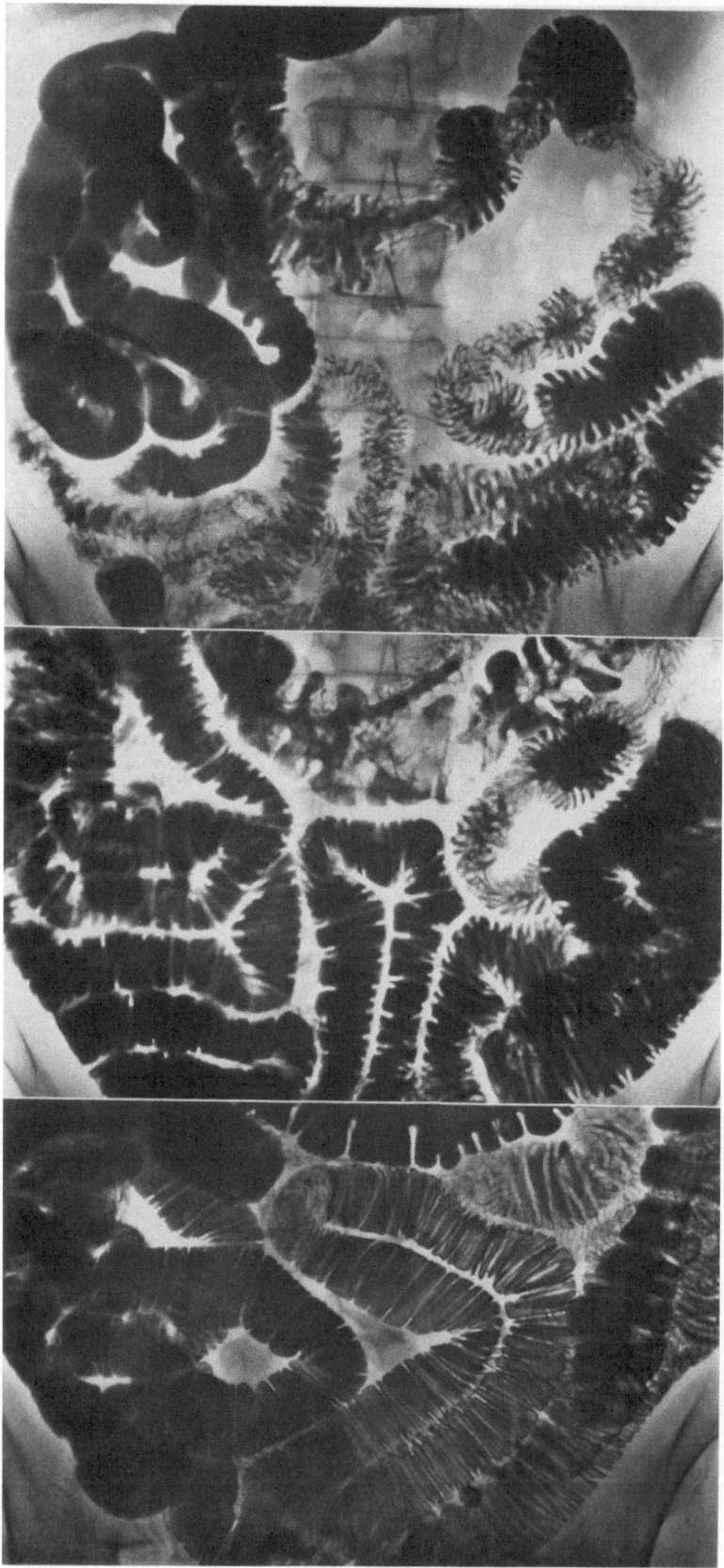

Fig. 65
Pat. 31: Third examination 6 weeks after
second. 600 ml Micropaque (s.g. 1.38)
through tube, followed by 600 ml water.
Definite abnormalities no longer seen.

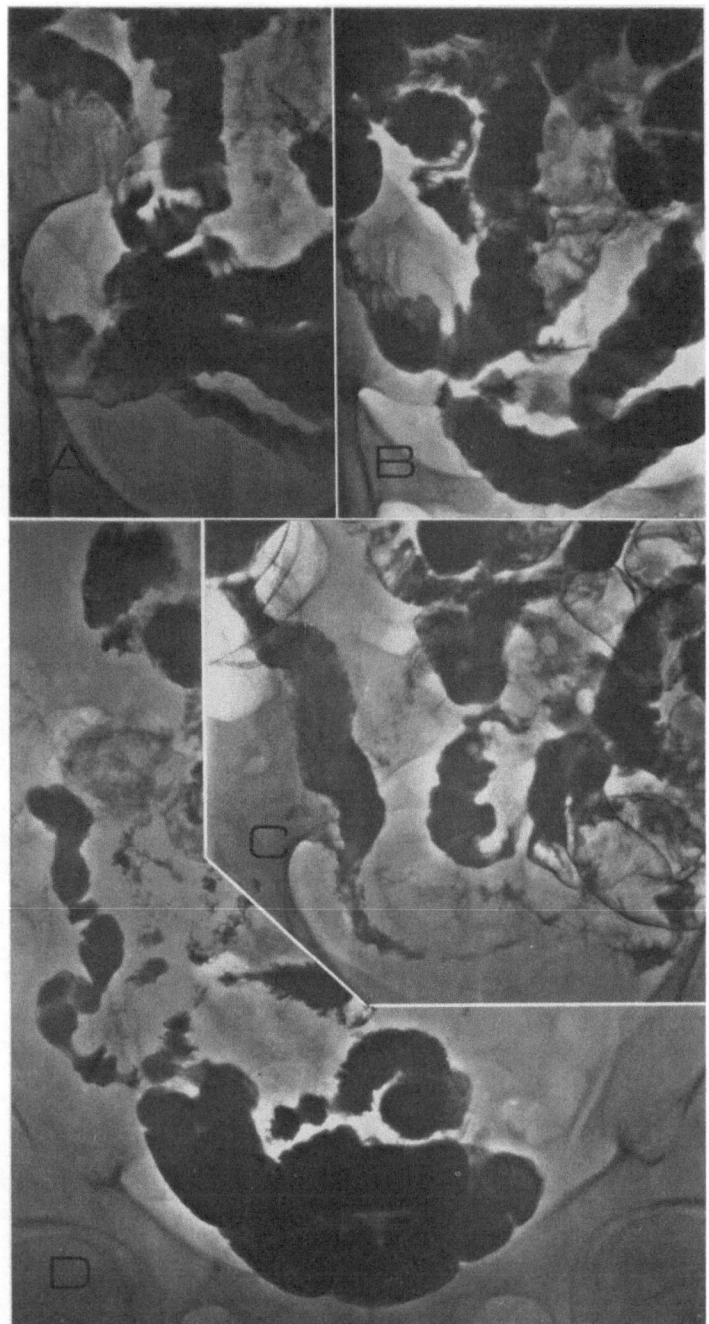

Fig. 66
Pat. 32: periodic abdominal pain for several years.
A, B, C: 600 ml Bario-dif (s.g. 1.23) administered
through tube in 12 min. Changes in mucosa in
distal ileum. Crohn's disease?
D: conv. examination 8 months before with 300 ml
Micr. AZL (s.g. 1.65). No abnormalities were found.

IX

The largest group consisted of 26 patients with vague abdominal complaints. For 10 patients, a conventional small intestine transit examination had been carried out previously; for 5 of these patients, Crohn's disease was suspected as a result of the examination after duodenal intubation. Our findings for these 5 patients were as follows.

Patient 32 showed highly pathological changes in the last ileum loop in the small pelvis over a length of approximately a half meter, suggesting Crohn's disease (figs. 66A-C). The conventional examination showed signs of disintegration of the contrast medium and therefore we could not find any mucosal changes (fig. 66D). This examination however had occurred 8 months earlier so that comparison is not really feasible although the patient's complaints have remained unchanged since that time.

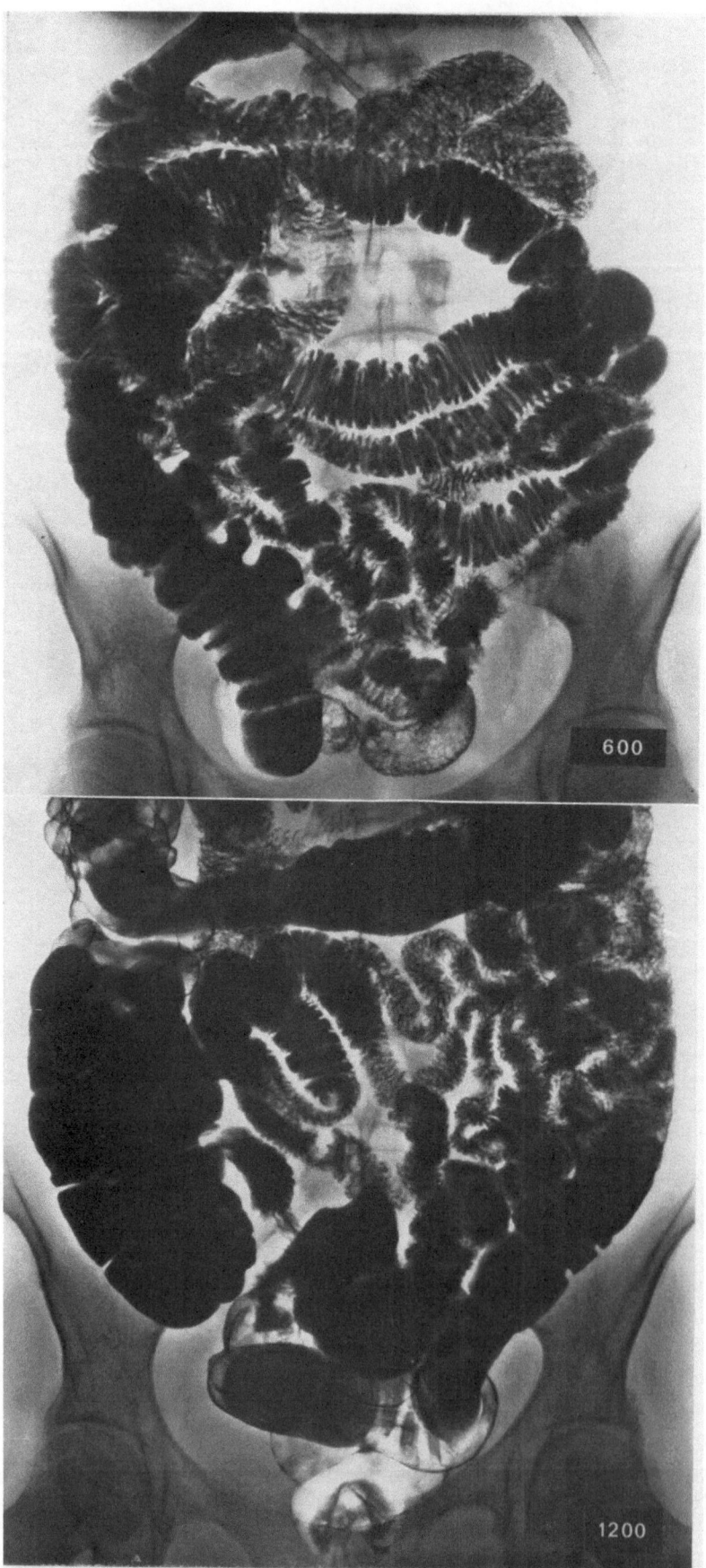

Fig. 67
Pat. 33: abdominal complaints
No abnormalities seen on survey
exposures after 600 and 1200 ml
Micropaque (s.g. 1.38) through tube.

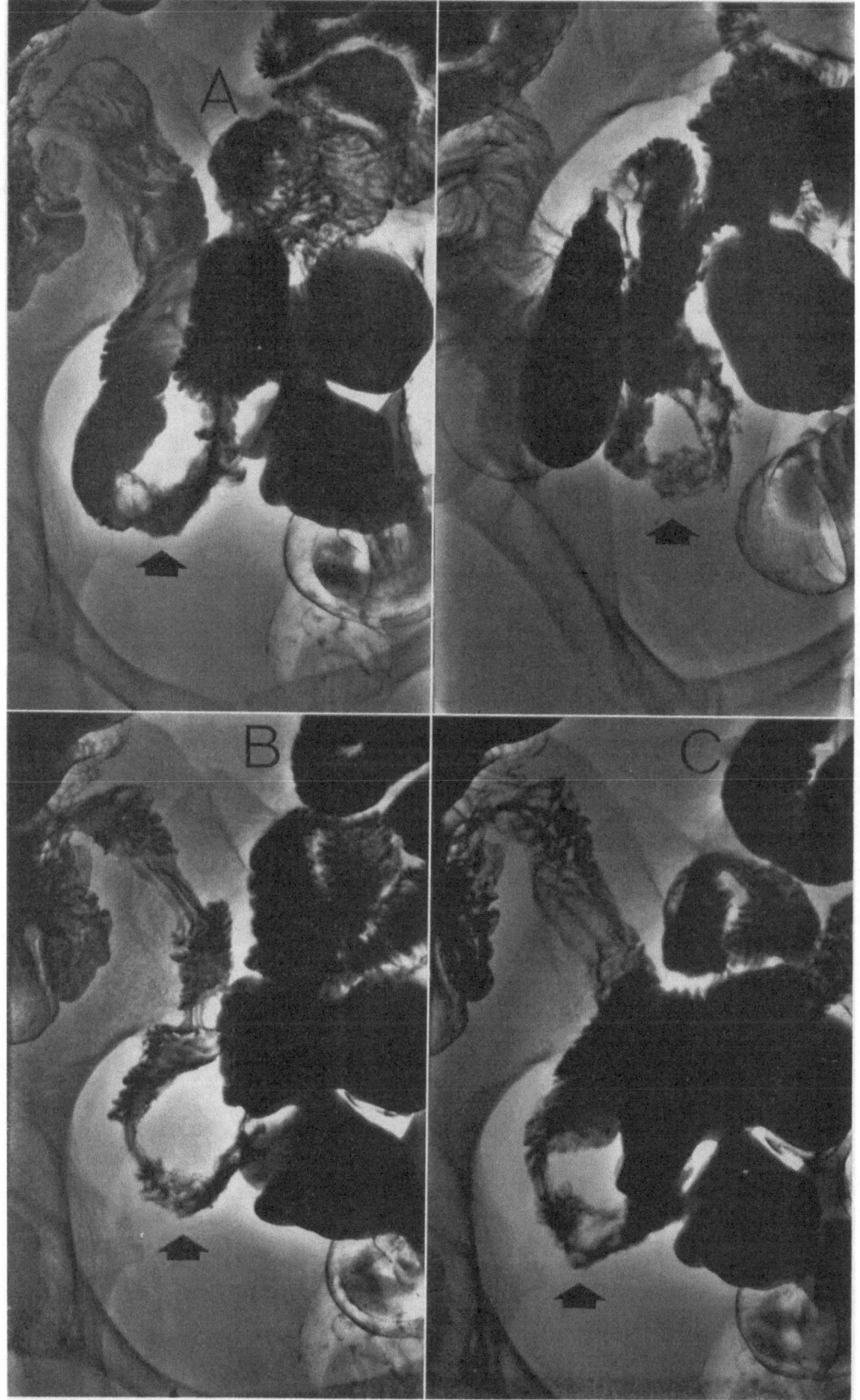

Fig. 68
Pat. 33: Spot film during compression after rectal air insufflation. Local abnormalities of the mucosa in a single ileum loop. Crohn's disease?

Patient 33 is a 29-year-old female. No special abnormalities were seen on the survey exposures taken with the infusion technique using 600 ml and 1200 ml contrast fluid (fig. 67). On the spot films taken during abdominal compression, changes in the mucosa can be seen in the ileum 15–20 cm before the valve of Bauhin over a length of several centimeters, suggesting Crohn's disease (fig. 68).

The conventional examination carried out elsewhere and lasting 5 hours revealed no abnormalities. The contrast fluid showed definite signs of disintegration during this examination (fig. 69).

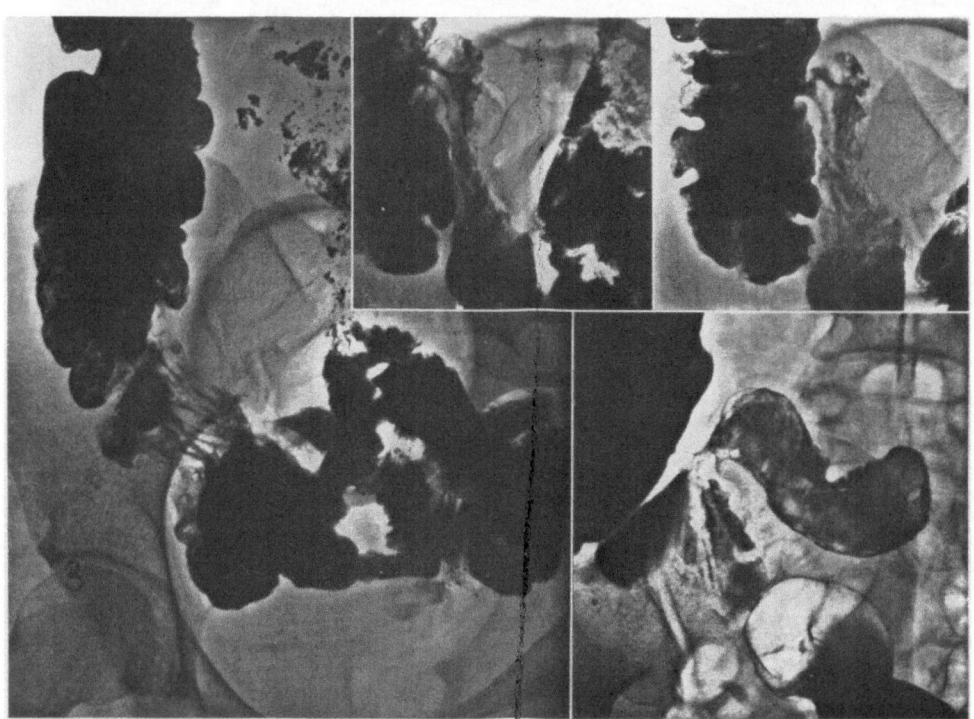

Fig. 69
Pat. 33: Conventional examination elsewhere 2 weeks earlier. No abnormalities found.

Patient 34 showed changes in the mucosa over a length of at least 30 cm of an ileum loop in the small pelvis, strongly suggesting Crohn's disease (fig. 70). The patient was examined several times by the conventional method. These examinations, which took place elsewhere, lasted quite long so that the x-rays show heavy segmentation of the contrast fluid (no films available). The x-rays of the examination after duodenal intubation of *patient 35* clearly show changes in the mucosa in the last 10 cm of the ileum, a stenosis in the region of the valve of Bauhin and some shriveling of the cecum (figs. 71A-C). These findings suggest Crohn's disease. It is striking that the conventional transit examination

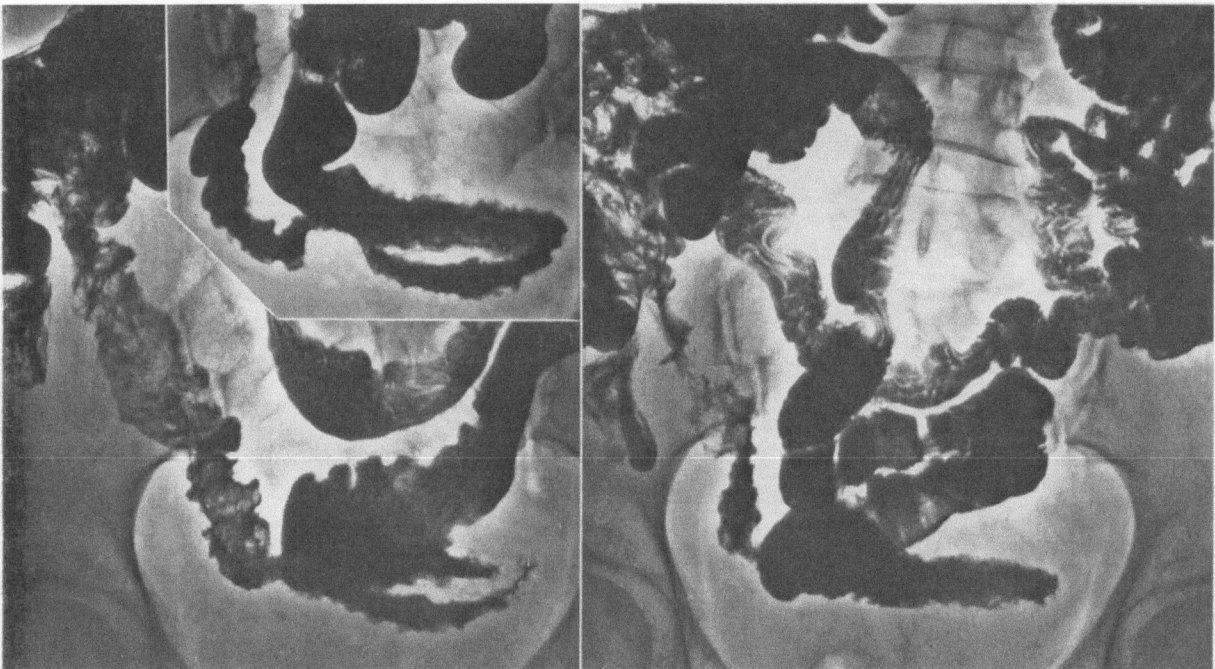

Fig. 70
Pat. 34: 600 ml Micropaque (s.g. 1.38) through tube in 10 min. Large section of ileum shows distinct changes in the mucosa. Crohn's disease?
The recent conventional examination revealed no abnormalities (heavy flocculation and segmentation).

6 years ago by our department also led to the suggested diagnosis of Crohn's disease. In my opinion however this diagnosis was highly speculative since the changes seen in the distal ileum during that examination could easily be ascribed to heavy disintegration of the contrast fluid (figs. 71D, E).

Patient 36 showed changes of the mucosa in the last 40 cm of the ileum in the infusion examination; Crohn's disease is suspected. There is also some shriveling of the cecum (fig. 72). The recent conventional transit examination, made elsewhere, lasted 6 hours. This examination also revealed mucosal changes in the distal ileum, although they are not as clearly seen (fig. 73).

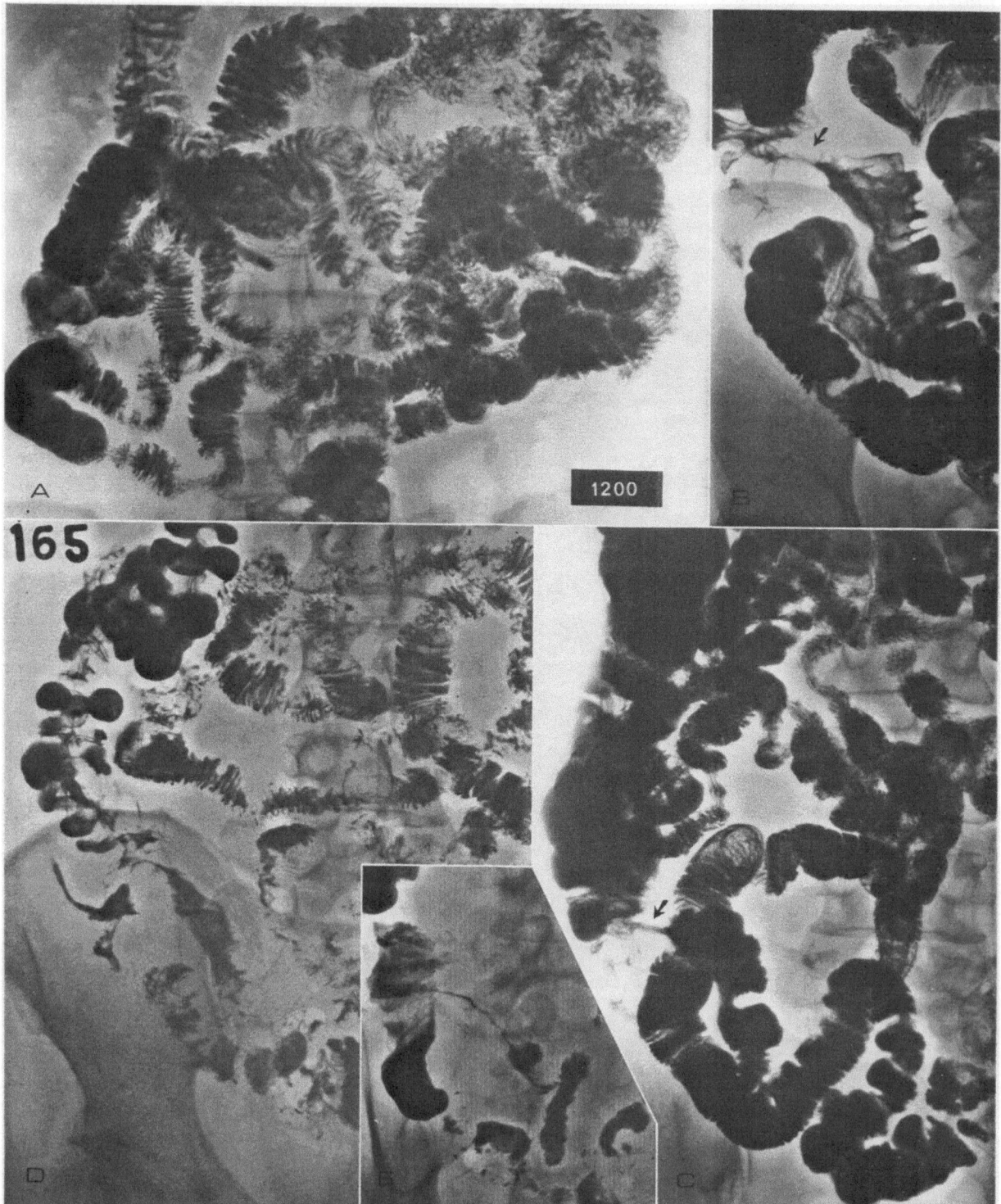

Fig. 71
Pat. 35: abdominal complaints for many years.
A, B, C: because of reflux into the stomach, 1200 ml Micr. AZL (s.g. 1.32) was administered through tube immediately. Stenosis in last 3 cm of ileum. Shriveled cecum. Crohn's disease?
D, E: conventional examination 6 years ago lasted 7 hours. Although Crohn's disease was suspected even then because of the string sign-like configuration in the distal ileum, this diagnosis must be considered speculative because of the advanced disintegration of the contrast fluid.

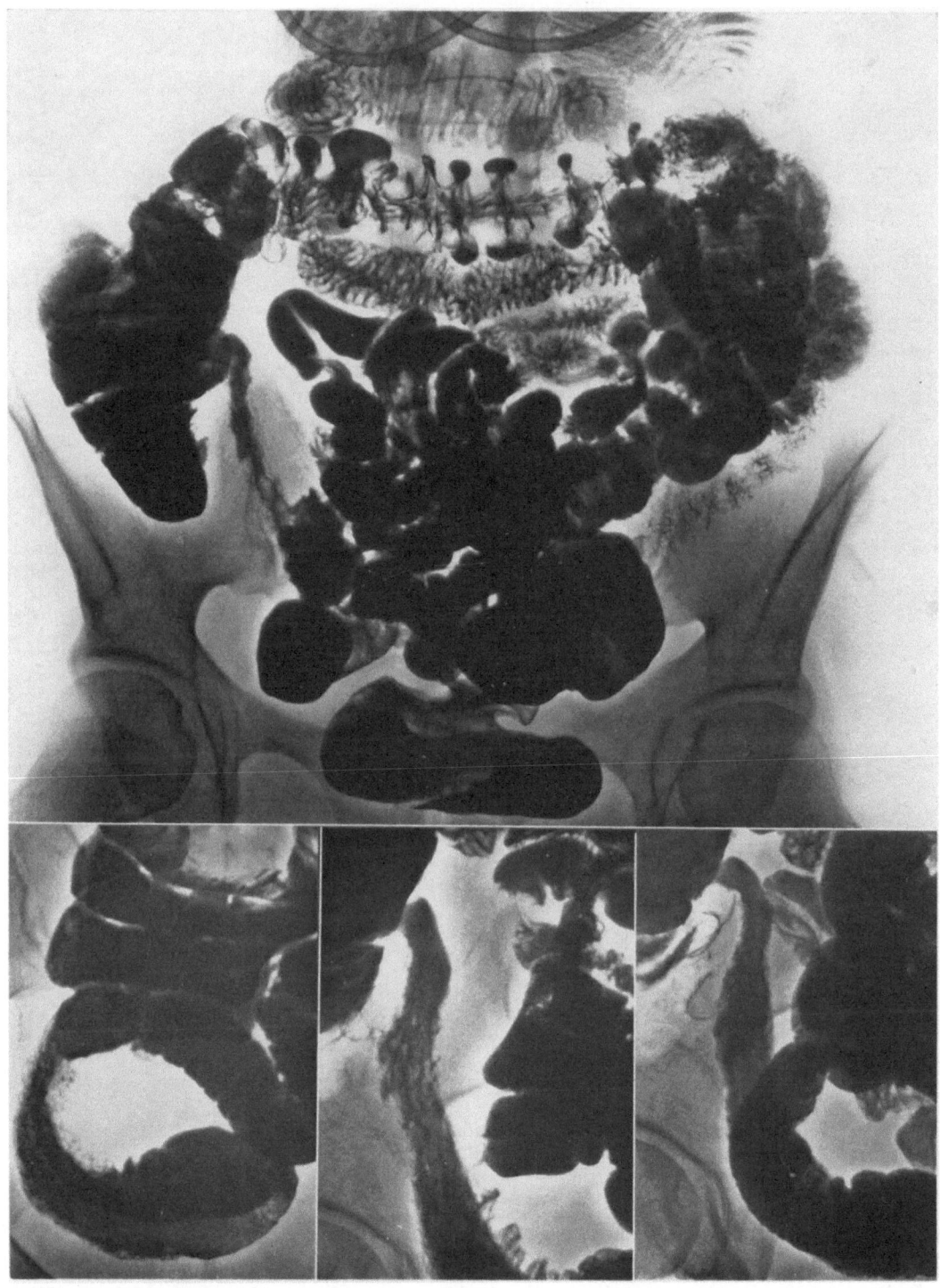

Fig. 72
Pat. 36: periodic abdominal complaints for last 4 years.
Duodenal infusion of 600 ml Micropaque (s.g. 1.38) followed by 300 ml water. Extensive abnormalities in distal ileum and shriveling of cecum. Crohn's disease?

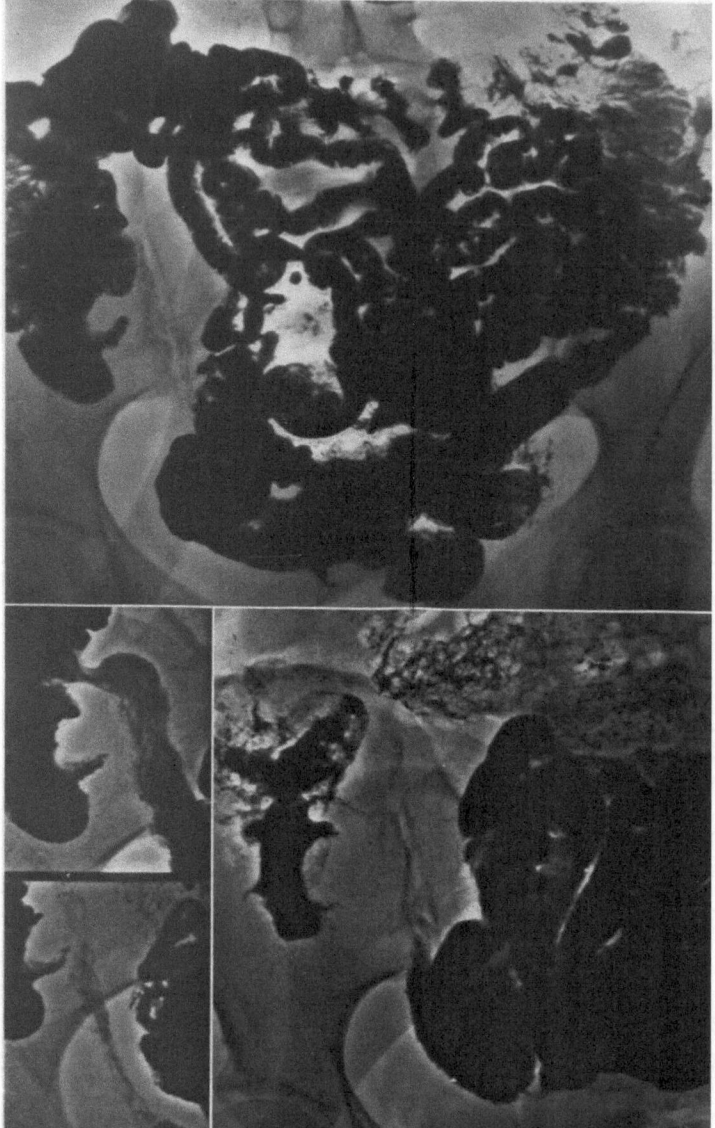

Fig. 73
Pat. 36: Recent conventional examination carried out elsewhere also
shows abnormalities in the distal ileum, although less clearly.

The following patients from this group are also worth mentioning.
In *patient 37*, the cecum, located quite deep in the small pelvis, was already visible by the end of the
5 minute infusion of 600 ml contrast medium. A very long appendix can be seen which reaches up-
ward and is fixed at its end (figs. 74A, B). In the upright position the cecum is suspended from the
appendix. It is possible that the patient's abdominal complaints can be explained by this phenomenon.

   Two weeks before the examination using the infusion technique, a conventional transit examination
took place with 300 ml of the same contrast medium and 30 ml Solcoray. The examination lasted
4 hours which led to dehydration and disintegration of the contrast fluid so that filling of the appendix
did not occur (figs. 74C, D).

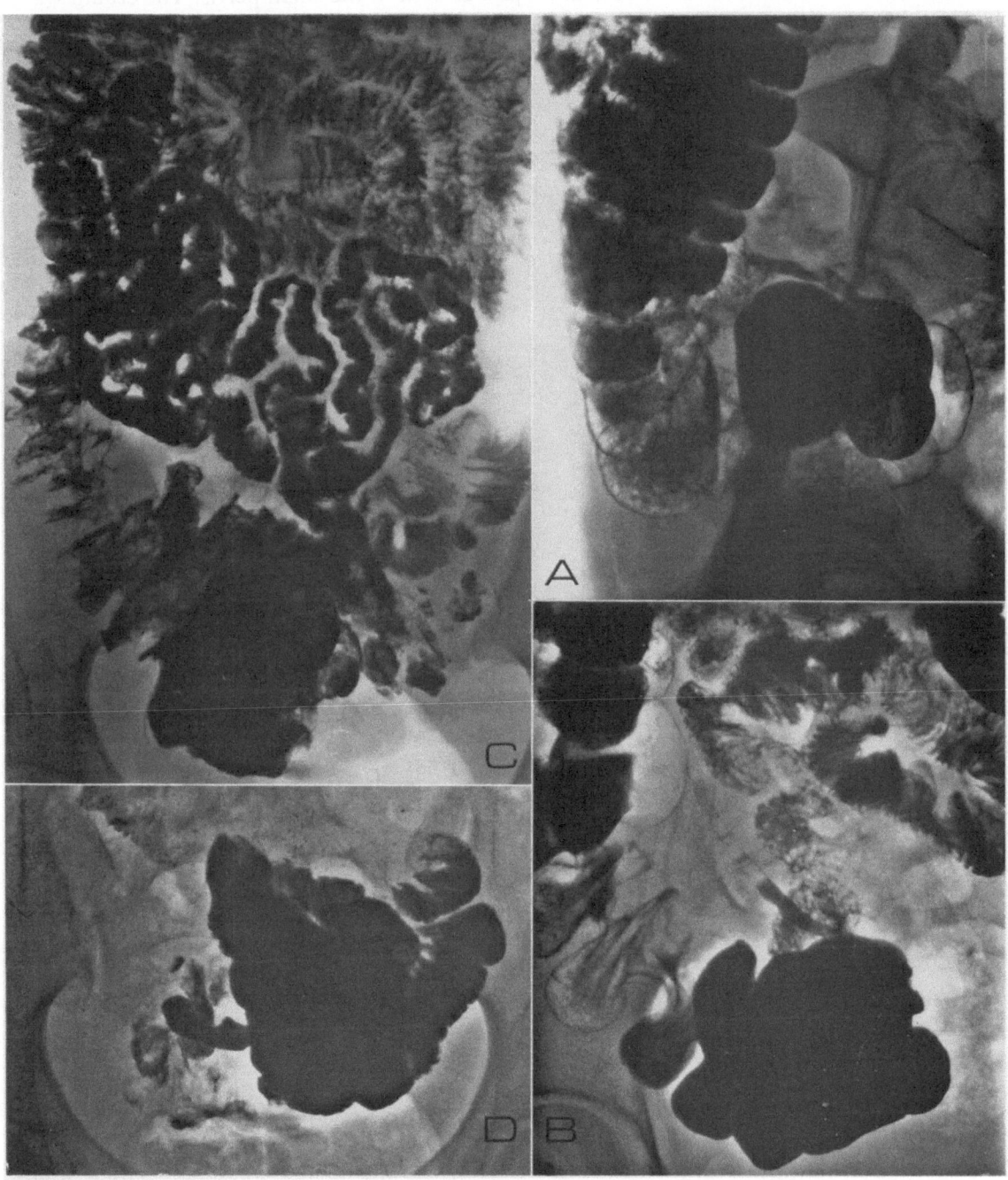

Fig. 74
Pat. 37:
A, B: 600 ml Micropaque (s.g. 1.26) through tube. Rectal air insufflation. Cecum very deep in small pelvis. Appendix
fixed at tip. Total examination time a half hour.
C, D: Conventional examination 2 weeks earlier lasted 6 hours. 300 ml Micropaque + 30 ml Solcoray. No useful
picture of cecum, appendix not filled (contrast fluid dehydration).

Patient 38: for the conventional technique, 300 ml Microbar AZL + 30 ml Solcoray were used, and 435 minutes later a compact mass of ileal loops was seen in the small pelvis. The cecum was not reached (fig. 75).

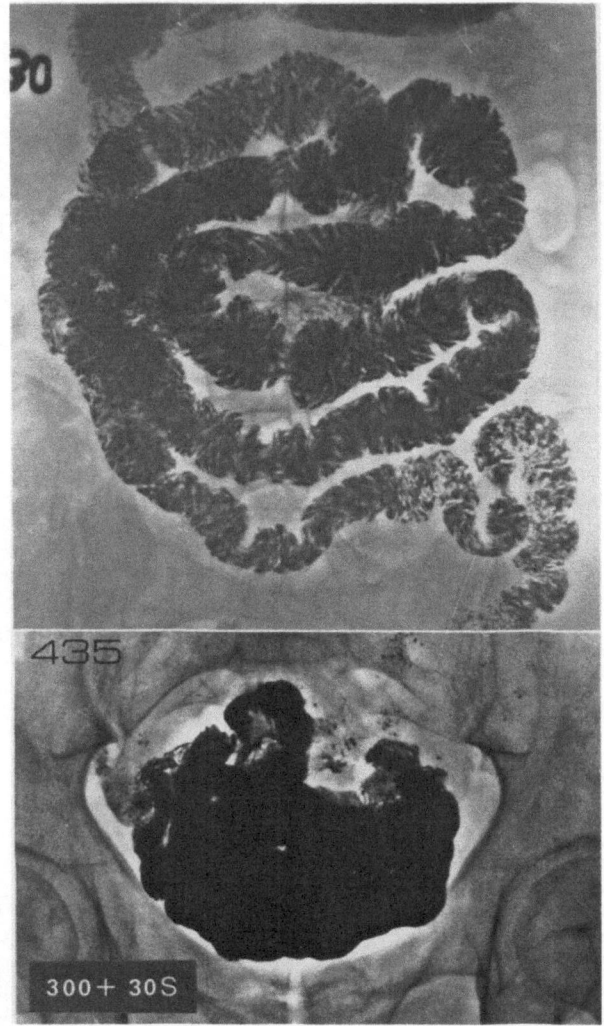

Fig. 75
Pat. 38: Conventional examination. 300 ml Micr. AZL (s.g. 1.32) + 30 ml Solcoray. Cecum not yet reached after 435 min.

One week later, an examination was carried out after duodenal intubation using 1200 ml of the same contrast fluid followed by 1200 ml water. Not until 45 minutes later was there good filling of the last ileum loop and the cecum (fig. 76). The x-rays show that in spite of the enormous quantities of contrast medium used, superposition of the intestinal loops is not annoying and that, even at the end of this examination, disintegration of the contrast fluid still occurs. Anatomical abnormalities were not found. The reason for the decreased peristalsis observed by fluoroscopy is not clear.

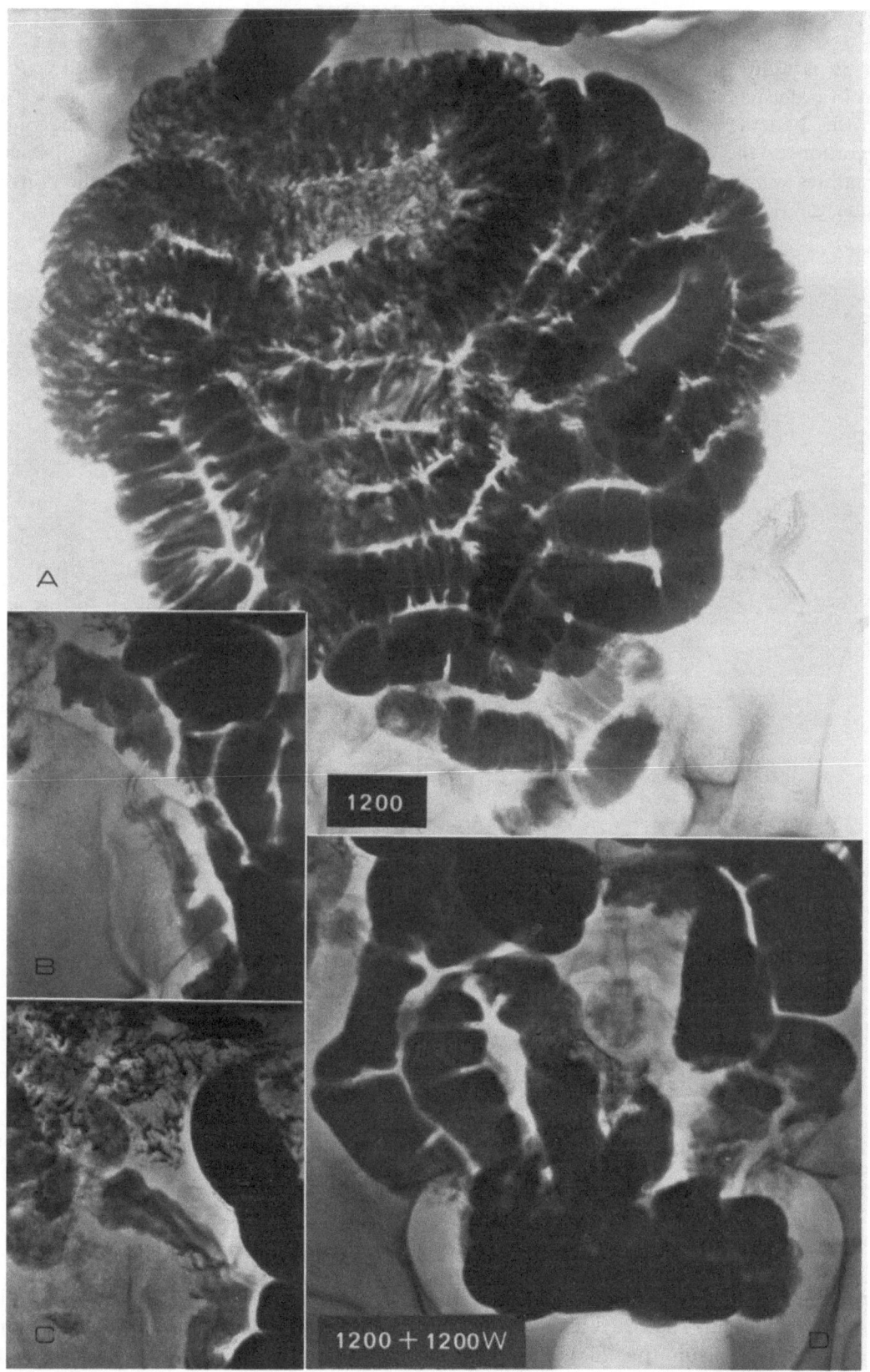

Fig. 76
Pat. 38: One week later, duodenal infusion of 1200 ml Micr. AZL (s.g. 1.32) + 1200 ml water and 20 ml Primperan (reflux into stomach). Now however distal ileum is seen. Total examination time 1 hour.

Patient 39 is quite similar to patient 38. Here too, 1200 ml contrast fluid and 1200 ml water had to be used in order to reach the cecum within a half hour. By fluoroscopy, reduced peristalsis was also seen in this patient. Annoying superposition of the intestinal loops did not occur and once again disintegration of the contrast fluid developed at the end of the examination (fig. 77). Anatomical abnormalities were not found. The patient had not been examined previously by the conventional technique.

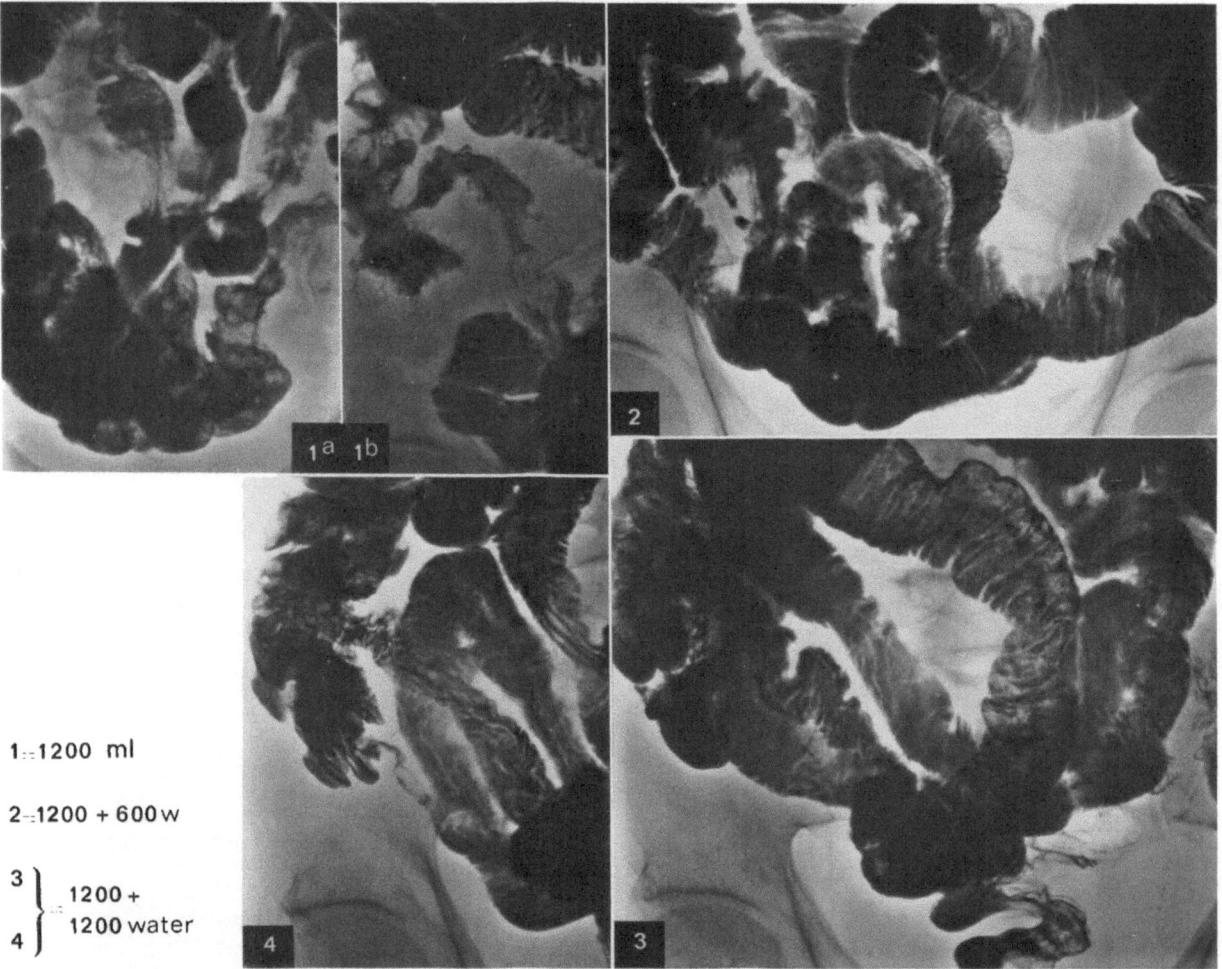

1 = 1200 ml

2 = 1200 + 600 w

3⎫
  ⎬ 1200 +
4⎭ 1200 water

Fig. 77
Pat. 39: In spite of administration of 1200 ml Micr. AZL and 1200 ml water through tube, the cecum was only reached after a half hour.
Exposure 3 shows beginning disintegration of barium suspension. No abnormalities can be seen.

Patient 40 underwent a conventional transit examination of the small intestine because of abdominal pain of unknown origin. The x-rays led to the diagnosis of Crohn's disease because of assumed mucosal changes in the distal ileum (fig. 78A). The colon examination 1 month later (fig. 78B), as well as the subsequent examination of the small intestine using the infusion technique (figs. 78C, 79), showed that there are no abnormalities in the distal ileum and that disintegration of the contrast fluid during the conventional transit examination led to an incorrect diagnosis.

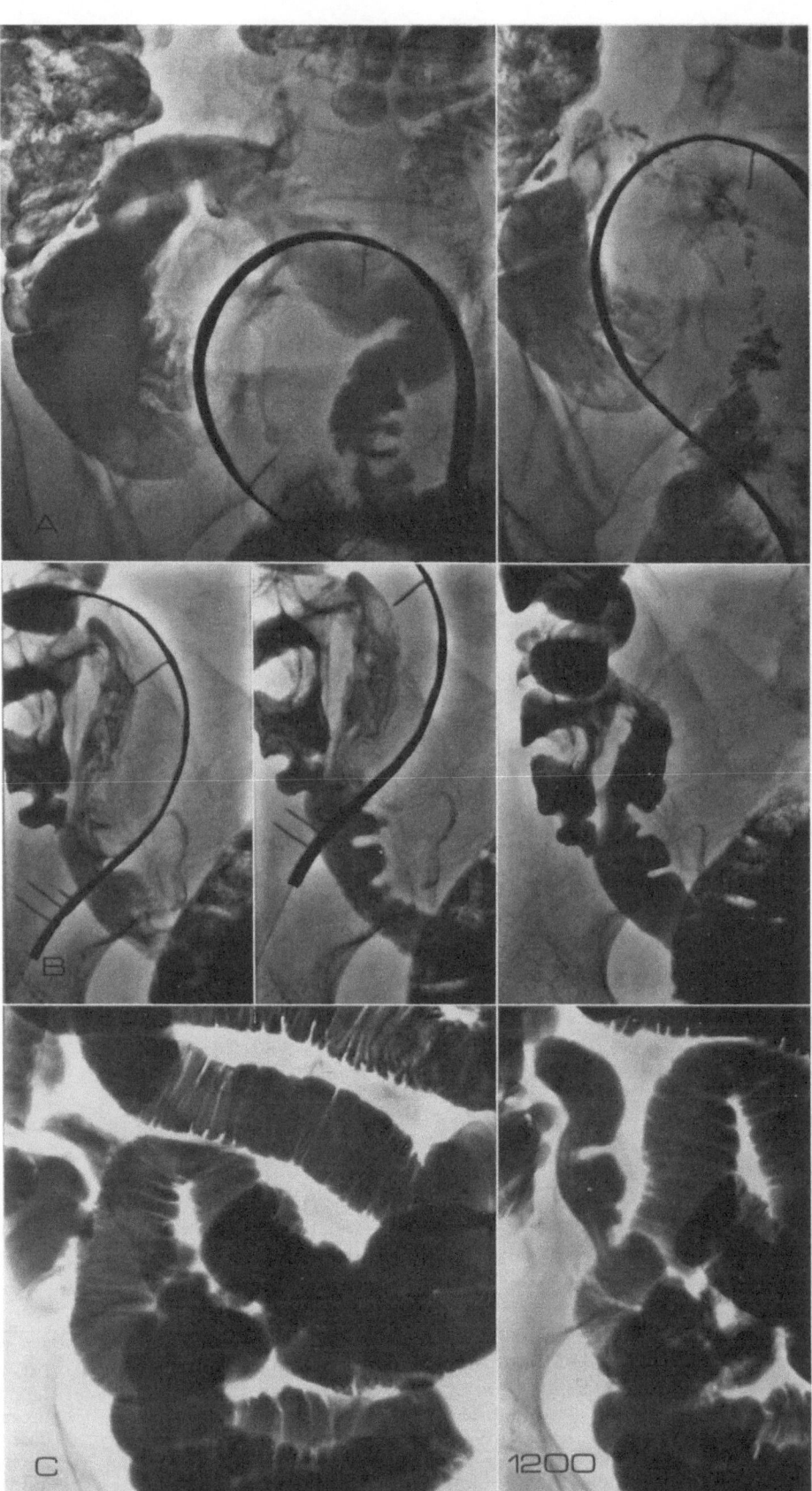

Fig. 78
Pat. 40: abdominal complaints of unknown origin.

A: conventional examination lasted 2.5 hours. Diagnosis of Crohn's disease in distal ileum; however disintegration of contrast fluid developed.

B: Colon examination 1 month later. No abnormalities.

C: Examination after duodenal intubation 1 year later. No abnormalities.

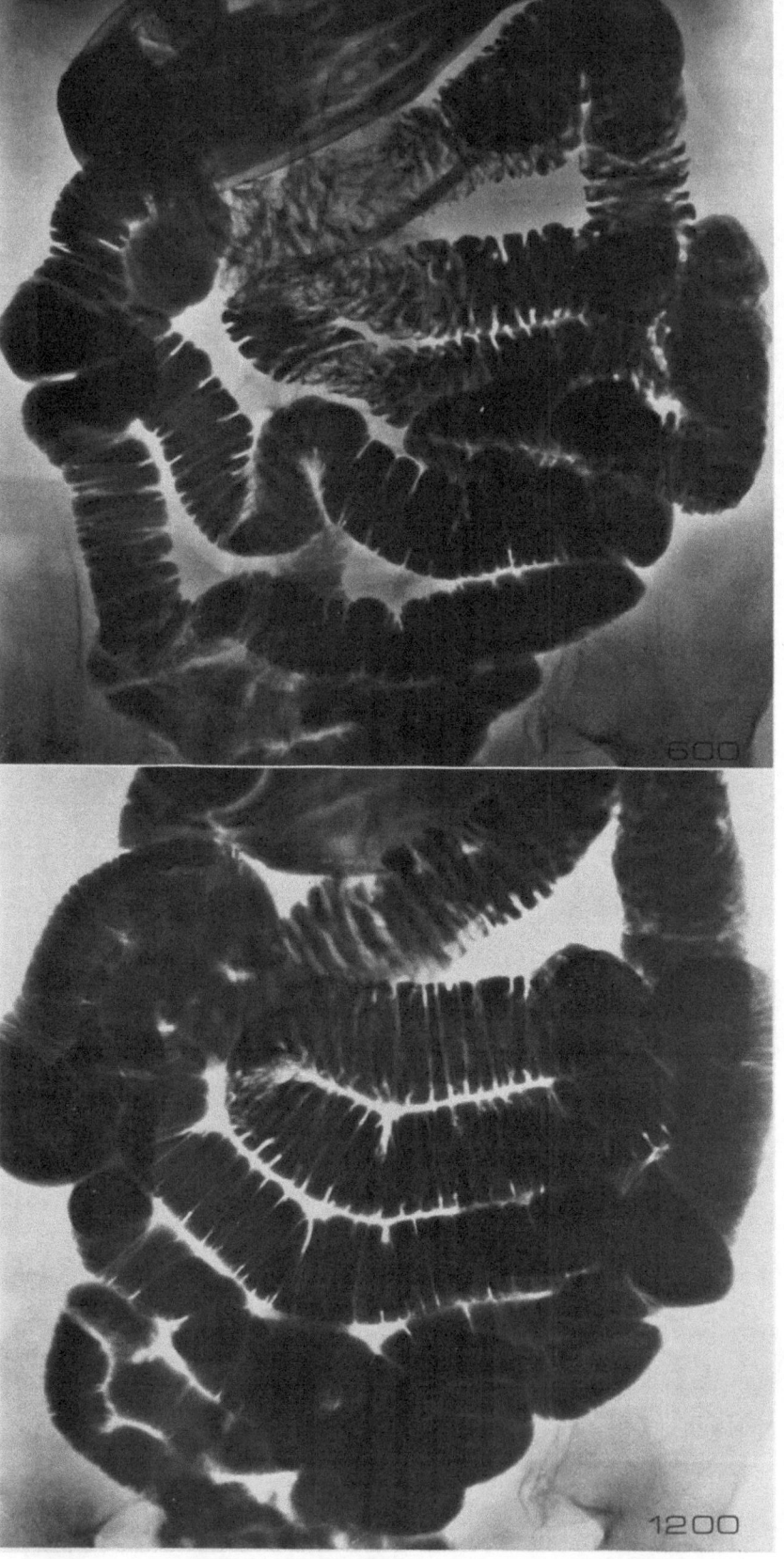

Fig. 79
Pat. 40: 600 ml Micropaque (s.g. 1.38) through duodenal tube. Because of reflux into stomach, 2nd dose of 600 ml. Superposition of intestinal loops usually increases less than would be expected with this supplementary dosage.

SUMMARY AND CONCLUSION

Although the examination of the small intestine has formed an important part of the daily 'menu' of the radiologist for the past 70 years, the results obtained still give little reason for satisfaction.

The use of drugs to accelerate passage not only shortened the duration of the examination considerably but in many cases also resulted in improved mucosal patterns.

The resistance of the contrast media to flocculation is highly variable but in general it has been improved by the addition of substances which increase the stability of the barium suspensions.

For some patients however the examination can still last many hours and finally may not be suited for interpretation after all because the contrast fluid has become dehydrated or has disintegrated into segment clumps. Other patients display such intense flocculation of the contrast fluid even during the initial stages of the examination that anatomical evaluation of the mucosa is often no longer possible during the rest of the examination. It is also very disappointing that smaller non-obstructing tumors in the small bowel are often not recognized by the radiologist, even when the contrast medium has retained its proper characteristics.

To a large extent the transit time is determined by the examination technique of the radiologist; the function of the pylorus musculature also has a greater influence on the transit time than various factors in the small intestine itself. The value attached to the observation of flocculation as well as transit times should therefore be highly relative since it can lead to incorrect conclusions.

The jejunum pictures can usually be interpreted more easily than those of the equally long ileum where most of the disorders which can be diagnosed radiologically are found. It is unfortunate that for free projection of the ileum loops, the patient must lie on his abdomen while on the other hand, the indispensible palpation and compression can only be carried out when he is lying on his back. The value of the examination of the small intestine is highly limited when an insufficient number of exposures are made. On the other hand it makes little sense to persist in continuously photographing segmented contrast clumps until the cecum is reached.

A good anatomical evaluation of the small intestine is only possible with a contrast medium which during the entire examination retains the same characteristics it had before being administered to the patient.

The manufacturers of contrast media have however not yet succeeded in producing a suspension which is practically insensitive to the diverse substances found in the digestive tract, in particular gastric acid.

BRAECKMAN and ZIMMER showed that in vitro flocculation of the contrast fluid increases with time according to a specific curve. It is also clear that administration of an excess of contrast medium will act as a buffer and the inconvenience of flocculation will be postponed.

As a result of fluid absorption, annoying thickening and dehydration of the contrast fluid occurs in the distal ileum, a process which also increases with time.

From the above, it can be concluded that the radiologist must try to quickly pass large amounts of the contrast fluid through the small intestine and that the damaging influence of gastric acid must be eliminated.

These requirements can only be satisfied by introducing the contrast medium directly into the duodenum through a tube. In this way, 600 ml can easily be administered in several minutes without inconveniencing the patient. In half the patients, the cecum has usually been reached by the time the infusion has ended. In many cases passage is slowed down if administration of the contrast medium is too slow or too fast. When it is too slow, the duodenal wall is not stretched enough to induce strong peristaltic waves; if it is too fast, reflux of the contrast fluid into the stomach often occurs. Peristalsis might decrease possibly owing to the entero-intestinal reflex mechanism.

For a conventional examination of the small intestine, passage through the pylorus can be stimulated by using an isotonic contrast medium. For infusion directly into the duodenum on the other hand, a hypotonic medium is more suitable because it stimulates contraction of the pylorus.

In the past, several radiologists administered the barium suspension through a tube directly into the duodenum. The earliest publication is by PESQUERA in 1929, the best known by SCHATZKI in 1943. LURA reported a total of 300 patients in 1951; PYGOTT and SCOTT-HARDEN described an improvement in the intubation technique in 1960.

Although the few authors who have reported on this technique for the examination of the small intestine were unanimously surprised by the excellent results obtained, this method has never been accepted for general use. Most likely this is due to the fact that intubation into the duodenum is often very time-consuming. The development of the Bilbao tube, based on the principle of the Seldinger catheter, has simplified duodenal intubation to such an extent that with experience it usually takes only several minutes; this factor can therefore no longer be seen as a disadvantage. The examination time has been shortened considerably and the number of intestinal loops seen per film is also greater than in a conventional transit examination. In addition the exposure of the contrast medium to the damaging influences of gastric and intestinal juices as well as dehydration in the ileum is greatly reduced. We have found therefore that when the infusion technique is used, it makes no difference whether a stable or an unstable contrast fluid is used. In the case of a slow transit, a supplementary dosage of contrast medium or water is the best means of enhancing peristalsis: administration of Sorbitol is never effective; Primperan is possibly useful only when reflux into the stomach has occurred.

The use of more than 900 ml contrast medium sometimes causes problems of superposition requiring an efficient compression technique, combined if necessary with oral or rectal gas insufflation. Another disadvantage of exceedingly high dosages can be that patients with a cardiac insufficiency could decompensate as a result. Bearing the dosage restrictions for these patients in mind, it can be stated that the anatomical evaluation of the small intestine by means of a roentgenological examination is much better when carried out in the manner described in this study than in any other manner. May the shortening of the examination time as well as the considerable improvement in diagnostic information stimulate the radiologist to pay more attention to the examination of the small intestine than is common at present.

BIBLIOGRAPHY

1. ABBOTT O; PENDERGRASS E. P. (1936) Intubation studies of the human small intestine. *Amer. J. Roentg.* **35**, 289–299.
2. ADAM A. (1932) Kontrastmittel und Innenwanddarstellung des Verdauungstraktes. *Fortschritte R.* **45/4**, 385–396.
3. ADLERSBERG D.; MARSHAK R. H.; COLCHER H.; DRACHMAN S. R.; FRIEDMAN A. I.; WANG C. I. (1954) The roentgenologic appearance of the small intestine in sprue. *Gastroenterology* **26/4**, 548–581.
4. ADOLPH W; TAPLIN G. V. (1950) Use of micropulverized barium sulfate in x-ray diagnosis. A preliminary report. *Radiology* **54/6**, 878–883.
5. ALEXANDER G. H; ALEXANDER R. E. (1950) The use of gastric mucin as a barium suspension medium. *Radiology* **54/6**, 875–877.
6. ALISTER MC. W. H.; ANDERSON S.; BLOOMBERG G. R; MARGULIS A. R. (1963) Lethal effects of tannic acid in the barium enema. Report of three fatalities and experimental studies. *Radiology* **80/5**, 765–773.
7. ANDERSON Ch. M.: ASTLEY R.; FRENCH J. M. and GERRARD J. W. (1952) The small intestine pattern in coeliac disease. *Brit. J. Radiol.* **25**, 526–530.
8. ARDRAN G. M.; FRENCH J. M; MUCKLOW E. H. (1950) Relationship of the nature of the opaque medium to small intestine radiographic pattern. *Brit. J. Radiol.* **23**, 697–702.
9. ARENS R. A; MESIROW S. D. (1937) Gastric mucosal relief. A modified sedimentation method, using a colloidally suspended bariumsulphate. *Radiology* **29**, 1–11.
10. ASTLEY R; FRENCH J. M. (1950) The small intestine pattern in normal children and in coeliac disease. Its relationship to the nature of the opaque medium. *Brit. J. Radiol.* **24**, 321–330.
11. BARCLAY A. E. (1938) The practical importance of mechanics in digestion. *Amer. J. Roentg.* **40**, 325–334.
12. BARDEN R. P.; THOMPSON W. D.; RAVDIN I. S.; FRANK I. L. (1938) The influence of the serum protein on the motility of the small intestine. *Surg. Gyn. Obst.* **66/5**, 819–821.
13. BEERSTECHER H. J. P. *De waarde van de ileo-rectale anastomose bij de chirurgische behandeling van de colitis ulcerosa.* Thesis, Leiden (to be published).
14. BENDICK A. J. (1954) *Diagnostic advances in gastrointestinal roentgenology.* New York.
15. BERGER G. (1968) Erfahrungen über die Verwendung von Visotrast in der Kinderklinik. (In der Magen-Darm-Diagnostik bei Kindern) *Dtsch. Gesundh.-Wes.* **23/8**, 356–360.
16. BERKOVITS L. JAVOR T. (1965) Über die Untersuchung des Dünndarms mit Enteramin. *Fortschritte R.* **103/1**, 60–62.
17. BERMAN C. Z; AVNET N. L. (1960) The use of water soluble urographic contrast media in paediatric. G.I. studies. *Brit. J. Radiol.* **33/386**, 92–97.
18. BILBAO M. K.; FRISCHE L. H.; DOTTER CH. T.; RÖSCH J. (1967) Hypotonic duodenography. *Radiology* **89**, 438–443.
19. BOURDON R; HUMMEL J. (1956) Basis de la radiologie du grêle. *J. Radiol. Electr.* **37/3–4**, 210–215.
20. BOUSLOG J. S. (1942) The normal stomach and small intestine in the infant. *Radiology* **39**, 253–260.
21. BOUSLOG J. S. (1937) The gastro-intestinal tract in children. *Radiology* **28**, 683–692.
22. BRAECKMAN P. (1947) Over suspensies met baryumsulfaat. *Pharm. Weekblad* **49/50**, 709–719.
23. BROWN F. O. (1959) On routine barium examination of the small bowel. *Lancet* **2** 530–533.
24. BROWN G. R. (1963) High-density barium-sulfate suspensions; an improved diagnostic medium. *Radiology* **81/5**, 839–846.
25. BUFFARD P. (1952) Le diagnostic des tumeurs de l'intestin grêle est-il possible dans le pratique radiologique quotidienne? *J. Radiol. Electr.* **33/1–2**, 64–66.

26. BUFFARD P.; CROZET L. (1952) Zur Dünndarmallergie. *Fortschritte R.* **76/4**, 497–507.

27. BUGYI B. (1955) Praktische Beiträge zur röntgenologischen Untersuchung der Verdauungsorgane. *Röntgenblätter* **8/4**, 107–111.

28. BULATAO E.; CARLSON A. J. (1924) Contributions to the physiology of the stomach. Influence of experimental changes in blood sugar level on gastric hunger contractions. *Amer. J. Physiol.* **69**, 107–115.

29. BURHENNE J. H.; VOGELAAR P.; ARKOFF R. S. (1966) Liver function studies in patients receiving enema's containing tannic acid. *Amer. J. Roentg.* **96/2**, 510–518.

30. BUSSCHER G. de (1950) Étude radiologique du grêle au cours de diverses affections. *Acta gastroent. belg.* **13/4**, 295–350.

31. CALDWELL W. L.; FLOCH M. H. (1963) Evaluation of the small bowel barium motor meal with emphasis on the effect of volume of barium suspensions ingested. *Radiology* **80/3**, 383–391.

32. CALDWELL W. L.; SWANSON V. L.; BAYLESS TH. M. (1965) The importance and reliability of the roentgenographic examination of the small bowel in patients with tropical sprue. *Radiology* **84/2**, 227–240.

33. CAMERON A. L. (1938 II) Primary malignancy of the jejunum and ileum. *Ann. of Surg.* **108**, 203–220.

34. CHAMBERLIN G. W. (1939 II) The roentgen anatomy of the small intestine. *J. Amer. med. Ass.* **113**, 1537–1541.

35. CLURE MC. C. W.; REYNOLDS L.; SCHWARTZ C. O. (1920) On the behavior of the pyloric sphincter in normal man. *Arch. int. Med.* **26**, 410–423.

36. COLE, the collaborators (1932) Findings observed in the gastro-intestinal tract. *Radiology* **18**, 886–941.

37. CROHN B. B.; GINZBURG L.; OPPENHEIMER G. D. (1932) Regional ileitis. A pathologic and clinical entity. *J. Amer. med. Ass.* **99/16**, 1323–1329.

38. CROWLEY R. T.; JOHNSTON CH. G. (1946) Physiological principles in intestinal obstruction. *Surg. Clin. N. Amer.* 1427–1439.

39. CUMMACK D. H. (1969) *Gastro-intestinal X-ray diagnosis*. Livingstone Ltd., Edinburgh.

40. CUMMINS A. J.; ALMY T. P. (1953) Studies on the relationship between motility and absorption in the human small intestine. *Gastroenterology* **23**, 179–190.

41. DEUCHER W. G. (1949) Über die Variabilität der Dünndarmschleimhaut. *Radiol. clin.* (Basel) **18/1**, 265–272.

42. DINER W. C. (1968) Small intestinal edema in cirrhosis; its disappearance with diuresis. *Radiology* **91**, 792–794.

43. DONATO H.; MAYO JR. H. W.; BARR L. H. (1954) The effect of peroral barium in partial obstruction of the small bowel. *Surgery* **35/5**, 719–723.

44. EMBRING G.; MATTSSON O. (1968) Barium contrast agents. *Acta radiol.* **7/NS diagn.** 3, 245–256.

45. EMBRING G.; MATTSSON O. (1966) An improved physiologic contrast medium for the alimentary tract. *Acta radiol.* **4/NS**, 105–109.

46. EPSTEIN B. S. (1957) The use of a water soluble contrast medium (Hypaque) for gastrointestinal roentgenography. *J. Amer. med. Ass.* **165**, 44–46.

47. ETTINGER A. J. H. (1949) Small intestinal pattern in sprue and similar deficiency diseases. *Amer. J. Roentg.* **61/5**, 658–670.

48. FABIAN M.; LAKOS A.; FEHER I. (1966) Passagebeschleunigende Methoden zur röntgenologischen Untersuchung des Darmtraktes. *Röntgenblätter* **19/1**, 58–64.

49. FIGIEL S. J.: FIGIEL L. S. (1964) Tumors of the terminal ileum. Diagnosis by retrograde filling during barium enema study. *Amer. J. Roentg.* **91**, 816–818.

50. FISCHER A. W. (1925) Uber die Röntgenuntersuchung des Dickdarms mit Hilfe einer Kombination von Lufteinblasung und Kontrasteinlauf. ('Kombinierte Methode'). *Archiv klin. Chir.* **134**, 209–269.

51. FLACH A. (1949) Vergleichende Untersuchungen über die Viscosität, Oberflächenspannung und Grenzflächenspannung verschiedener Kontrastmittel. *Röntgenblätter* **2/6**, 303–310.

52. FLOCH M. H.; CALDWELL W. L.; SHEEHY T. W. (1962) A histopathologic basis for the interpretation of small bowel roentgenography in tropical sprue. *Amer. J. Roentg.* **87/4**, 709–716.

53. FORSSELL G. (1923) Studies of the mechanism of movement of the mucous membrane of the digestive tract. *Amer. J. Roentg.* **2**, 87–104.

54. FORSSELL G. (1939) Role of autonomous movements of the gastrointestinal mucous membrane in digestion. *Amer. J. Roentg.* **41**, 145–165.

55. FOUBERT F.; ROBERT F. (1951) Intérêt d'un nouveau support de produit de contraste dans le radiodiagnostic digestif: la Carboxy-Méthyl-Cellulose. *J. Radiol. Electr.* **32**, 925.

56 FRAZER A. C.; FRENCH J. M.; THOMPSON M. D. (1949) Radiographic studies showing the induction of a segmentation pattern in the small intestine in normal human subjects. *Brit. J. Radiol.* **22/255**, 123–136.

57. FRENCH J. M. (1950) Further studies in the radiology of the small intestine. *Gastroenterologia* (Basel) **76/6**, 343–345.

58. FRIEDENBERG M. J.; ALISTER MC. W. H.; MARGULIS A. R. (1962) Roentgen study of the small bowel in adults and children with neostigmine. *Amer. J. Roentg.* **88/4**, 693–701.

59. FRIEDMAN J. (1954) Roentgen studies of the effects on the small intestine from emotional disturbances. *Amer. J. Roentg.* **72**, 367–379.

60. FRIEDMAN J.; RIGLER L. G. (1950) A method of double-contrast roentgen examination of the small intestine. *Radiology* **54**, 365–379.

61. FRIK K.; BLÜHBAUM TH. (1928) Eine neue Anwendungsart der Kolloide in der Röntgendiagnostik. *Fortschritte R.* **38/6**, 1111–1120.

62. FRIMAN-DAHL J. (1954) The administration of barium orally in acute obstruction; advantages and risks. *Acta Radiol.* **42**, 285–295.

63. FURNEMONT E. (1966) L'utilisation du Sorbitol dans l'exploration radiologique du tractus intestinal. *Acta gastroent. belg.* 24/8–9, 779–790.

64. GERSHON-COHEN J.; SHAY H. (1939) Barium enteroclysis. A method for the direct immediate examination of the small intestine by single and double contrast techniques. *Amer. J. Roentg.* **42/3**, 456–458.

65. GERSHON-COHEN J.; SHAY H.; FELS S. S. (1940) The relation of meal temperature to gastric motility and secretion. *Amer. J. Roentg.* **43/2**, 237–242.

66. GERSHON-COHEN J.; SHAY H.; FELS S. S. (1938) Experimental studies on gastric physiology in man. The influence of osmotic pressure changes of salt and sugar solutions on pyloric action and gastric emptying in the normal and operated stomach. *Amer. J. Roentg.* **40**, 335–343.

67. GERSHON-COHEN J.; SHAY H. (1937) Experimental studies on gastric physiology in man. A study of pyloric control. The rôle of milk and cream in the normal and in subjects with quiescent duodenal ulcer. *Amer. J. Roentg.* **38**, 427–446.

68. GIANTURCO C. (1950) Fast radiological visceral survey. *Radiology* **54**, 59–64.

69. GIRAND M.; BRET P.; PINET F.; ROCHE P. (1951) L'examen radiologique du grêle par transit accéléré. *J. Radiol. Electr.* **32/7–8**, 583–595.

70. GLASER F. H.; KÖLLING H. L. (1967) Beitrag zur peroralen Magen-Darm-Diagnostik mit Bariumsulfat-Amidotrizoat-Gemischen. *Radiol. diagn.* (Berl.) **8**, 13–22.

71. GOIN L. S. (1952) Some obscure factors in the production of unusual small bowel patterns. *Radiology* **59/2**, 177–184.

72. GOLDEN R. (1951) Advances in gastro-enterological radiology 1937–1950. *Brit. J. Radiol.* **24**, 237–245.

73. GOLDEN R. (1959) Technical factors in the roentgen examination of the small intestine. *Amer. J. Roentg.* **82/6**, 965–972.

74. GOLDEN R. (1959) *Radiologic examination of the small intestine.* second ed. J.B. Lippincott, Philadelphia.

75. GOLDEN R. (1941) Abnormalities of the small intestine in nutritional disturbances. *Radiology* **36**, 262–286.

76. GOLDEN R. (1950) Some clinical problems in small intestinal physiology. *Brit. J. Radiol.* **23**, 390–409.

77. GOOD A. (1963) Tumors of the small intestine. *Amer. J. Roentg.* **89**, 685–705.

78. GREENSPON E. A.; LENTINO W. (1960) Retrograde enterography. A new method for the roentgenologic study of the small bowel. *Amer. J. Roentg.* **83/5**, 909–919.

79. GRIER T.; MILLER; KARR W. G. (1936) Intubation studies of the human small intestine. The influence of variations in the reaction and the motility of the stomach contents on the reaction and the motility of the intestinal contents. *Amer. J. Roentg.* **35**, 300–305.

80. HANAFEE W.; WEINER M. (1967) External guided passage of an intestinal intubation tube. *Radiology* **89**, 1100–1102.

81. HARRIS P. D.; NEUHAUSER E. B. D.; GERTH R. (1964) The osmotic effect of water soluble contrast media on circulating plasma volume. *Amer. J. Roentg.* **91/3**, 694–698.

82. HECHT G. (1934) *Heubners Handbuch der experimentellen Pharmakologie* **8**, 97. Springer, Berlin.

83. HEITZMAN R. E.; BERNE A. S. (1961) Roentgen examination of the cecum and proximal ascending colon with ingested barium. *Radiology* **76**, 415–421.

84. HENDERSON S. G. (1942) The gastrointestinal tract in the healthy newborn infant. *Amer. J. Roentg.* **48**, 302–335.

85. HENDERSON N. P. (1944) The value of the opaque enema and its modifications. *Brit. J. Radiol.* **17**, 140–149.

86. HIGHMAN J. H. (1964) Urinary excretion as a sign of intestinal perforation. *Brit. J. Radiol.* **37**, 697–700.

87. HIRSCH J.; AHRENS E.; BLANKENHORN D. H. (1956) Measurement of the human intestinal length in vivo and some causes of variation. *Gastroenterology* **31**, 274–285.

88. HODGES F. J.; RUNDLESS R. W.; HANELIN J. (1947) I. Roentgenologic study of the small intestine. Neoplastic and inflammatory diseases. *Radiology* **49**, 587–602.
    II. Roentgenologic study of the small intestine. Dysfunction associated with neurologic diseases. *Radiology* **49**, 659–673.

89. HOLT J. F.; LYONS R. H.; NELIGH R. B.; NOE G. K.; HODGES F. J. (1947) x-ray signs of altered alimentary function following autonomic blockade with tetraethylammonium. *Radiology* **49/5**, 603–610.

90. HOLZKNECHT G. (1931) *Handbuch der theoretischen und klinischen Röntgenkunde.* Wien.

91. HOWARTH F. H.; COCKEL R.; ROPER B. W.; HAWKINS C. F. (1969) The effect of metoclopramide upon gastric motility and its value in barium progress meals. *Clin. radiol.* **20**, 294–300.

92. HUDAK A. (1951) Le transit accéléré du grêle. *Radiol. clin.* (Basel) **20/3**, 148–154.

93. HÜPCHER N. (1961) Het gebruik van bariumsulfaatsuspensies, in het bijzonder tylosebarium in de tractus digestivus. *J. belge Radiol.* **44/2**, 161–169.

94. JAMES W. B.; HUME R. (1968) Action of metoclopramide on gastric emptying and small bowel transit time. *Gut* **9**, 203–205.

95. JANOWER M. L.; ROBBINS L. L.; TOMCHIK F. S.; WEYLMAN W. T. (1965) Tannic acid and the barium enema. *Radiology* **85/5**, 887–894.

96. JEFFRIES G. H.; WESER E.; SLEISINGER M. H. (1964) Progress in gastroenterology. Malabsorption. *Gastroenterology* **46**, 434–466.

97. JOHNSTON C. G.; RAVDIN I. S. (1935, I) Action of glucose on emptying of stomach. Effect of varying concentrations in both normal stomachs and after various gastric operations. *Amer. Surg.* **101**, 500–505.

98. JOLLASSE. (1907) Zur Motilitätsprüfung des Magens durch Röntgenstrahlen. *Fortschritte R.* **11**, 47–53.

99. JONES G. E.; CHALECKE W. E.; DEC J.; SCHILLING J. A.; RAMSEY G. H.; ROBERTSON H. D.; STRAIN W. H. (1947) Jodinated organic compounds as contrast media for radiographic diagnosis. Studies on tetraiodophthalimidoethanol as a medium for gastrointestinal visualization. *Radiology* **49/2**, 143–151.

100. KAESTLE. (1907) Bolus alba und Bismutum subnitricum, eine für die röntgenologische Untersuchung des Magen-Darmkanals brauchbare Mischung. *Fortschritte R.* **11**, 266–271.

101. KNOX R. (1919) *Radiography and radio-therapeutics.* E. and C. Black Ltd., London.

102. KANTOR J. L. (1939) The roentgendiagnosis of idiopathic steatorrhea and allied conditions. Practical value of the 'Moulage sign'. *Amer. J. Roentg.* **41/5**, 758–778.

103. KING C. E.; ARNOLD L. (1922) The activities of the intestinal mucosal motor mechanism. *Amer. J. Physiol.* **59**, 97–121.

104. KIRSH I. E. (1956) Motility of the small intestine with non-flocculating medium; A review of 173 roentgen examinations. *Gastroenterology* **31**, 251–260.

105. KIRSH I. E.; SPELLBERG M. A. (1953) Examination of small intestine with carboxymethylcellulose. *Radiology* **60**, 701–707.

106. KNOEFEL P. K.; DAVIS L. A.; PILLA L. A. (1956) Agglomeration of barium sulfate and roentgen visualisation of the gastric mucosa. *Radiology* **67/1**, 87–91.

107. KORPASSY B.; HORVAI R.; KOLTAY M. (1951) On the absorption of tannic acid from the gastrointestinal tract. *Arch. int. Pharmacodyn.* **88**, 368–377.

108. KUNZ B.; LEMM M.; HAUBACH D. (1965) Die Verwendung von „Visotrast 370" in der Magen-Darm Diagnostik. *Dtsch. Gesundh.-Wes.* **20/13**, 593–595.

109. LAFONTAINE A. (1965) Danger de l'acide tannique utilisé en lavement. *J. belge Radiol.* **48/5**, 551–555.

110. LAREN MC. J. W. (1960) *Modern trends in diagnostic radiology. Third series. Examination of the small bowei* by W. G. Scott Harden 84–87. Butterworths, London.

111. LÄSER S. (1966) Verbesserungen der Eigenschaften von Bariumsulfatsuspensionen für die Magen-Darm-Passage durch Zusatz von Polysaccharidlösungen. *Schweiz. med. Wschr.* **96/19**, 633–638.

112. LAWS J. W.; NEALE G. (1966) Radiological diagnosis of disaccharidase deficiency. *Lancet* **II**, 139–143.

113. LAWS J. W.; PITMAN R. G. (1960) The radiological investigation of malabsorption syndromes. *Brit. J. Radiol.* **33**, 211–228.

114. LAWS J. W.; SHAWDON H.; BOOTH C. C.; STEWART J. S. (1963) Correlation of radiological and histological findings in idiopathic steatorrhea. *Brit. med. J.* **May**, 1311–1314.

115. LEB A. (1951) Eine Röntgen-Digestionsprüfung. Die Röntgenuntersuchung des resezierten Magens mit Eiweiss- und Fett- Bariumkernen. *Fortschritte R.* **75**, 106–116.

116. LEDOUX-LEBARD G. (1968) Histoire de la radiologie du tube digestif. *Gaz. med. Fr.* **75/2**, 209–216.

117. LEHNER H. H.; MÄRKI W.; ZIMMER E. A. (1948–49) Ueber ein neues Barium-Kontrastmittel, zugleich ein Beitrag zur Prüfung solcher Substanzen. *Gastroenterologia* (Basel) **74/4**, 193–208.

118. LENZ H. (1962) Weitere Untersuchungen zur Funktionsanalyse der Dünndarmperistaltik. *Fortschritte R.* **97/2**, 147–159.

119. LENZ H. (1962) Die Segmentationsbewegungen des Ileums im Röntgenkinobild. *Fortschritte R.* **97/2**, 159–168.

120. LENZ H.; KREPPEL E. (1965) Röntgenkinematographische Untersuchungen über das Verhalten der Dünndarmmotorik bei der Katze unter Prostigmin, Pilocarpin und Arecolin. *Fortschritte R.* **102/3**, 268–277.

121. LESSMAN F. P.; LILIENFELD R. M. (1959) Gastrografin as water soluble medium in roentgenexamination of the G.I. tract. *Acta radiol.* **51/3**, 170–178.

122. LETTERS K.; GAUL M. (1951) Neue Untersuchungen zur Charakterisierung von Röntgenkontrastmittel für Magen und Darm. *Fortschritte R.* **74/2**, 229–234.

123. LIERE E. J. v.; NORTHUYS D. W.; CLIFFORD S. J. (1946) The effect of glucose on the motility of the stomach and small intestine. *Gastroenterology* 7, 218–223.

124. LÖNNERBLAD L. (1951) Transit time through the small intestine. A roentgenologic study on normal variability. *Acta radiol.* suppl. **88**.

125. LURA A. (1951) Radiology of the small intestine. Enema of the small intestine with special emphasis on the diagnosis of tumours. *Brit. J. Radiol.* **24/281**, 264–271.

126. MAGNUSSON W. (1931) On meteorism in pyelography and on the passage of gas through the small intestine. *Acta radiol.* **12**, 552–561.

127. MANECKE H; SCHMIDT F. W. (1962) Die Magen-Darm-Passage mit Karion. *Fortschritte R.* **97/2**, 142–146.

128. MARETIĆ Z.; HOMADOVSKI J.; RAZBOJNIKOV S.; BRECEVIC V. (1957) Barium poisoning. Ein Beitrag zur Kenntnis von Vergiftung mit Barium. *Med. Klin.* **52/45**, 1950–1953.

129. MARGULIS A. R. (1967) Some new approaches to the examination of the gastro intestinal tract. *Amer. J. Roentg.* **101**, 265–286.

130. MARGULIS A. R.; MANDELSTAM P. (1961) The use of parenteral neostigmine in the roentgen study of the small bowel. *Radiology* 76, 223–229.

131. MARGULIS A. R.; BURHENNE H. J. (1967) *Alimentary tract roentgenology.* C. V. Mosby Company, St. Louis.

132. MARSHAK R. H. (1961) Roentgen findings in lesions of the small bowel. *Amer. J. dig. Dis.* 6, 1084–1114.

133. MARSHAK R. H.; LINDNER A. E. (1970) *Radiology of the small intestine.* W. B. Saunders Company, Philadelphia.

134. MARSHAK R. H.; LINDNER A. E. (1966) Malabsorption syndrome. *Seminars Roentg.* 1/2, 138–177.

135. MARSHAK R. H.; KHILNANI M.; ELIASOPH J.; WOLF B. S. (1967) Intestinal edema. *Amer. J. Roentg.* **101/2**, 379–387.

136. MARSHAK R. H.; WOLF B. S.; COHEN N.; JANOWITZ H. D. (1961) Proteinlosing disorders of the gastrointestinal tract: Roentgen features. *Radiology* 77/6, 893–905.

137. MARSHAK R. H.; WOLF B. S.; ADLERSBERG D. (1954) Roentgenstudies of the small intestine in sprue. *Amer. J. Roentg.* **72**, 380–400.

138. MARSHAK R. H.; FRIEDMAN A. J.; WOLF B. S.; CROHN B. B. (1951) Roentgen findings in ileo-jejunitis. *Gastroenterology* 19/3, 383–408.

139. MARTEL W.; HODGES F. J. (1959) The small intestine in Whipple's disease. *Amer. J. Roentg.* 81/4, 623–636.

140. MATTSSON O.; PERMAN G.; LAGERLÖF H. (1960) The small intestine transit time with a physiologic contrast medium. *Acta radiol.* **54**, 334–344.

141. MELLINK J. H. (1961) Radiophysical aspects of the use of contrast substances in radiogdiagnosis. *J. belge Radiol.* 44/2, 107–126.

142. MENVILLE L. J.; ANÉ J. N. (1932) An x-ray study of the passage of different foodstuffs through the small intestine of man. *Radiology* 18, 783–786.

143. MILLER R. E.; BRAHME F. (1969) Large amounts of orally administered barium for obstruction of the small intestine. *Surg. Gyn. Obst.* **129/6**, 1185–1188.

144. MILLER R. E.; MILLER W. J. (1966) Inflammatory lesions of the small bowel. Complete reflux small bowel examination. *Amer. J. Gastroent.* **45**, 40–49.

145. MILLER R. E. (1965) Barium sulfate suspensions. *Radiology* 84/2, 241–251.

146. MILLER R. E. (1965) Complete reflux small bowel examination. *Radiology* 84/3, 457–463.

147. MORETON R. D.; YATES CH. W. (1950) The double-contrast study of the colon. A comparative study of barium sulfate preparations. *Radiology* 54, 541–547.

148. MORI P. A.; BARRETT H. A. (1962) A sign of intestinal perforation. *Radiology* 79/3, 401–407.

149. MORRISON B. O.; HALEY T. J.; PAYZANT A. R.; GENTNER G. A.; PAGON-CARLO J. (1959) Use of Hypaque as contrast medium in G.I. examination. *Amer. J. Gastroent.* 31/4. 398–407.

150. MORTON J. L. (1961) Notes on a small bowel examination. *Amer. J. Roentg.* 86/1, 76–85.

151. MÜLLER J. H. A. (1968) Die Röntgendiagnostik des Dünndarms mit Neostigmine. *Dtsch. Gesundh.-Wes.* 23/9, 391–397.

152. MUNTEAU E. (1951) Experimentelle Grundlagen einer röntgenologischen Eiweiss Digestionsprüfung. *Radiol. Austr.* 4, 187–199.

153. MURRAY J. P. (1966) Buscopan in diagnostic radiology of the alimentary tract. *Brit. J. Radiol.* 39/458, 102–111.

154. NAUMANN W. (1948) *Funktionelle Dünndarmdiagnostik im Röntgenbild.* Thieme, Stuttgart.

155. NELSON S. W.; CHRISTOFORIDIS A. J. (1967) The use of barium sulfate suspensions in the study of suspected mechanical obstruction of the small intestine. *Amer. J. Roentg.* **101**, 367–378.

156. NELSON S. W.; CHRISTOFORIDIS A. J.; ROENIGK W. J. (1965) Dangers and fallibilities of jodinated radiopaque media in obstruction of the small bowel. *Amer. J. Surgery* 109, 546–559.

157. NICE CH. M. (1963) Roentgenographic pattern and motility in small bowel studies. *Radiology* 80, 39–45.

158. PAJEWSKI M.; ITZCHAK Y.; PROFIS A. (1970) The double contrast examination of the small intestine. Preliminary communication of a new technique. *Clin. radiol.* **21**, 83–86.

159. PANSDORF H. (1937) Die Fraktionierte Dünndarmfüllung und ihre klinische Bedeutung. *Fortschritte R.* **56**, 627–634.

160. PATTERSON D. E.; RAD M.; DAVID R.; BAKER S. J. (1965) Radiodiagnostic problems in malabsorption. *Brit. J. Radiol.* **38/447**, 181–191.

161. PENDERGRASS E. P. (1936) The small intestine. *J. Amer. med. Ass.* **107/23**, 1859–1861.

162. PENDERGRASS E.; RAVDIN I. S.; JOHNSTON C. G.; HODES P. J. (1936) The effect of foods and various pathologic states on the gastric emptying and the small intestinal pattern. *Radiology* **26**, 651–662.

163. PEREZ C. A.; FRIEDENBERG M. J. (1967) Comparison of carboxy-methyl-cellulose, tannic-acid and no additive in barium examinations of the colon. *Amer. J. Roentg.* **99/1**, 98–105.

164. PESQUERA G. S. (1929) A method for the direct visualization of lesions in the small intestines. *Amer. J. Roentg.* **22/3**, 254–257.

165. PIRK F.; STÁHLAVSKÁ A.; CERNÁ M. (1967) Vergleich der Eigenschaften einiger Bariumkontrastmittel verschiedener Herkunft. *Radiol. diagn.* (Berl.) **8/6**, 773–780.

166. PIRK F.; VULTERINOVÁ M. (1964) The x-ray picture of the small intestine and impaired absorption. *Radiol. clin.* (Basel) **33/4**, 249–267.

167. POCK-STEEN O. C.; LORENZEN J. (1968) Gluten-intolerance and food allergy. Clinical signs and radiological changes of the small intestine. *Radiol. clin.* (Basel) **37/2**, 65–78.

168. PORCHER P.; CAROLI J. (1957) Un accélérateur inattendu du transit intestinal (grêle et colon). *Arch. Mal. Apper. dig.* **46/7-8**, 663–665.

169. PORTIS S. A. (1941) The clinical significance of the roentgenological findings of the small intestine. *Radiology* **37**, 289–293.

170. PREGER L.; AMBERG J. R. (1967) Sweet diarrhea. Roentgen diagnosis of disaccharidase deficiency. *Amer. J. Roentg.* **101/2**, 287–295.

171. PRÉVÔT R. (1940) Ergebnisse röntgenologischer Dünndarmstudien unter besonderer Berücksichtigung der Morphologie. *Fortschritte R.* **62/2**, 341–388.

172. PYGOTT F. (1958) *Modern trends in gastroenterology.* Butterworth, London.

173. PYGOTT F.; STREET D. F.; SHELLSHEAR M. F.; RHODES C. J. (1960) Radiological investigation of the small intestine by small bowel enema technique. *Gut* **1**, 366–370.

174. RAIFORD TH. S. (1931) Tumors of the small intestine. Their diagnosis, with special reference to the x-ray appearance. *Radiology* **16**, 253–270.

175. REIDELL H. (1937) Vergleichende Untersuchungen an Magen-Darmkontrastmitteln. *Fortschritte R.* **56**, 653–662.

176. REINHARDT K. (1960) Untersuchungen über den Wert einer Sorbitolbeimischung zum Bariumbrei für die Röntgendarstellung des Darmtraktes. *Fortschritte R.* **92**, 78–84.

177. REINHARDT J. F.; BARRY W. F. (1962) Scleroderma of the small bowel. *Amer. J. Roentg.* **88/4**, 687–692.

178. REYNOLDS L.; MACY I. G.; HUNSCHER H.; OLSON M. B. (1940) The gastro-intestinal response of average, healthy children to test meals of barium in milk, cream, meat and carbohydrate media. *Amer. J. Roentg.* **43/4**, 517–532.

179. RICE R. P.; ROUFAIL W. M.; REEVES R. J. (1967) The roentgen diagnosis of Whipple's disease (Intestinal lipodystrophy). *Radiology* **88**, 295–301.

180. RIEDER H. (1904–05) Beiträge zur Topographie des Magen-Darmkanals beim lebenden Menschen, nebst Untersuchungen über den zeitlichen Ablauf der Verdauung. *Fortschritte R.* **8**, 141–172.

181. ROBINSON D.; LEVENE J. M. (1958) Oral Renografin: A new contrast medium for gastrointestinal tract. *Amer. J. Roentg.* **80**, 79–81.

182. ROSEN R. S.; JACOBSON G. (1965) Visible urinary tract excretion following oral administration of water-soluble contrast-media. *Radiology* **84/6**, 1031–1032.

183. RUBIN R. J.; OSTRUM B. J.; DEX W. J. (1960) Water-soluble contrast media. Their use in the diagnosis of obstructive gastrointestinal disease. *Arch. Surg.* **80**, 495–500.

184. SACK G. M. (1963) Die orale Schnellpassage des Darms. *Fortschritte R.* **99/3**, 337–342.

185. SCHATZKI R. (1943) Small intestinal enema. *Amer. J. Roentg.* **50/6**, 743–751.

186. SCHÖNBAUER E. (1955) Mitteilung über die Verwendung von Baridol in der Magen-Darmdiagnostik. *Röntgenblätter* **8**, 8–15.

187. SCOTT-HARDEN W. G.; HAMILTON H. A. R.; MC CALL SMITH S. (1961) Radiological investigation of the small intestine. *Gut* **2**, 316–322.

188. SEARS A. D.; HAWKINS J.; KILGORE B. B.; MILLER J. E. (1964) Plain roentgenographic findings in drug induced intramural hematoma of the small bowel. *Amer. J. Roentg.* **91**, 808–813.

189. SEIJSS R. (1961) High kV technique for gastro-intestinal diagnosis. *Röntgenblätter* **14/2**, 54–56.

190. SHAY H.; GERSHON-COHEN J. (1934–6) Experimental studies in gastric physiology in man. A study of pyloric control. The rôles of acid and alkali. *Surg. Gyn. Obst.* **L VIII,** 935–955.

191. SHEHADI W. H. (1963) Studies of the colon and small intestines with water-soluble jodinated contrast media. *Amer. J. Roentg.* **89/4,** 740–751.

192. SHEHADI W. H. (1960) Orally administered water-soluble jodinated contrast media. *Amer. J. Roentg.* **83,** 933–941.

193. SHUFFLEBARGER H. E.; KNOEFEL P. K.; TELFORD J.; DAVIS L. A.; PIRKEY E. L. (1953–5) Some factors influencing the roentgen visualization of the mucosal pattern of the gastrointestinal tract. *Radiology* **61,** 801–805.

194. SIDAWAY M. E. (1964) Use of water-soluble contrast medium in paediatric radiology. *Clin. radiol.* **15/2,** 132–138.

195. SINCLAIR D. J.; BUIST T. A. S. (1966) Instrumental and technical notes. Water contrast barium enema using methyl cellulose. *Brit. J. Radiol.* **39/459,** 228–232.

196. SLOAN R. D.; BROCK J. W.; FANT W. M. (1961) Non-strangulating distal ileal obstruction. The rôle of hydration. An experimental study correlating pathologic and radiologic findings. *Radiology* **76,** 407–414.

197. SLOAN R. D. (1957) The mucosal pattern of the mesenteric small intestine; an anatomic study. *Amer. J. Roentg.* **77/4,** 651–669.

198. SNELL A. M.; CAMP J. D. (1934) Chronic idiopathic steatorrhea. Roentgenologic observations. *Arch. int. Med.* **53,** 615–629.

199. SÖVÉNYI E.; VARRÓ V. (1959) Uber eine neue Methode zur Röntgenuntersuchung des Dünndarms. *Fortschritte R.* **91/2,** 269–270.

200. SPENCER R. P. (1961) Microvilli and intestinal surface area: An evaluation. *Gastroenterology* **41,** 313–314.

201. STACY G. S.; LOOP J. W. (1964) Unusual small bowel diseases. Methods and observations. *Amer. J. Roentg.* **92/5,** 1072–1079.

202. STECKEN A.; RICHTER K.; WEISS U. (1961) Zur Kontrastmitteldarstellung des Magen-Darm-Traktes. Ergebnisse von 117 Untersuchungen mit Gastrografin und Gastrografin-Bariumsulfat Gemischen. *Fortschritte R.* **95/2,** 172–188.

203. STEINBACH H. L.; BURHENNE J. (1962) Performing the barium enema: Equipment, preparation and contrast medium. *Amer. J. Roentg.* **87,** 644–654.

204. SUSSMAN M. L.; WACHTEL E. (1943) Factors concerned in the abnormal distribution of barium in the small bowel. *Radiology* **40,** 128–138.

205. SWISCHUK L. E.; WELSH J. D. (1968) Roentgenographic mucosal patterns in the 'malabsorption syndrome'. A scheme for diagnosis. *Amer. J. dig. Dis.* **13/1,** 59–78.

206. TACHEV T.; HADJIDEKOV G.; NEDKOVA-BRATANOVA N.; IJANEV S. (1967) Radiologic stigmata of allergic enteropathies. *Acta gastroent. belg.* **30/3,** 209–224.

207. THORNER R. S. (1955) The effect of exclusion of the bile upon gastrointestinal motility. *Amer. J. Roentg.* **74,** 1096–1122.

208. TOSCH R. (1961) Untersuchungen über die Resorption von J 131 markiertem Gastrografin aus dem Magen-Darm kanal. *Fortschritte R.* **95/2,** 189–192.

209. UNDERHILL B. M. L. (1955) Intestinal length in man. *Brit. med. J.* **4950,** 1243–1246.

210. VEST B.; MARGULIS A. R. (1962) Roentgen diagnosis of postoperative ileus-obstruction. *Surg. Gyn. Obst.* **115,** 421–427.

211. WEEL J. G. A. V.; WOUTERS J. O. (1963) Het meten van röntgencontraststoffen 'in vitro' door middel van röntgen-stralen. *J. belge Radiol.* **46/5,** 481–489.

212. WEIGEN J. F.; PENDERGRASS E. P.; RAVDIN I. S.; MACHELLA T. E. (1952) A roentgen study of the effect of total pancreatectomie on the stomach and small intestine of the dog. *Radiology* **59,** 92–102.

213. WEINTRAUB S.; WILLIAMS R. G. (1949) A rapid method of roentgenologic examination of the small intestine. *Amer. J. Roentg.* **61,** 45–55.

214. WELTZ G. A. (1937) Der kranke Dünndarm im Röntgenbild. *Fortschritte R.* **55,** 20–40.

215. WILSON J. P. (1967) Surface area of the small intestine in man. *Gut* **8,** 618–621.

216. WOOLDMAN E. E. (1938) Barium sulphate suspension in colloidal Aluminium hydroxyde. An improved contrast medium for the roentgenographic diagnosis of gastro-intestinal lesions. *Amer. J. Roentg.* **40,** 705–707.

217. WOLF B. S.; FAEGENBURG D. H. (1963) Progress in gastroenterology. *Gastroenterology* **44,** 886–899.

218. WOLF B. S. (1959) Functional aspects of gastro-intestinal radiology. *Surg. Clin. N. Amer.* **39/5,** 1431–1449.

219. YOUMANS W. B. (1944) The intestino-intestinal inhibitory reflex. *Gastroenterology* **3,** 114–118.

220. ZASLON J.; PORTNER J. H.; COHEN E. A.; KREMENS V.; BERGER S. M. (1961) Complete small intestinal obstruction in the absence of positive roentgen findings. *Amer. J. Gastroent.* **35/2,** 122–126.

221. ZBORALSKE F.; BESSOLO R. J. (1967) Metastatic carcinoma of the mesentery and gut. *Radiology* **88,** 302–310.

222. ZBORALSKE F.; HARRIS P. A.; RIEGELMAN S.; RAMBO O. N.; MARGULIS A. R. (1966) Toxity studies on tannic acid administered by enema. Studies on the retention of enemas in humans. Review and conclusions. *Amer. J. Roentg.* **96/2**, 505–509.

223. ZIMMER E. A. (1954) Die Röntgenologie des Dünndarms. *Gastroenterologia* (Basel) **70**, 113–171.

224. ZIMMER E. A. (1948–49) Barium 'Wander'. A new contrastmedium with special advantages in examination of the gastro-intestinal tract. *Gastroenterologia* (Basel) **74/4**, 208–224.

225. ZIMMER E. A. (1951) Radiology of the small intestine. Studies on contrastmedia for the x-ray examination of the gastro-intestinal tract. *Brit. J. Radiol.* **24**, 245–251.

226. ZOLLNER S. (1937) Physiologische Schwankungen in der Motorik des Dünndarms. *Fortschritte R.* **56**, 644–649.